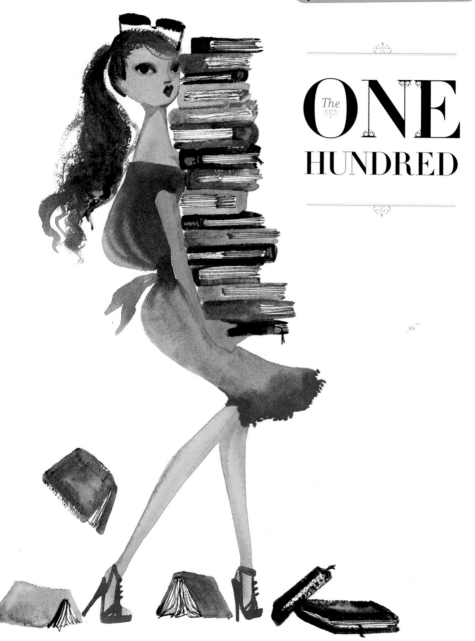

The ONE HUNDRED

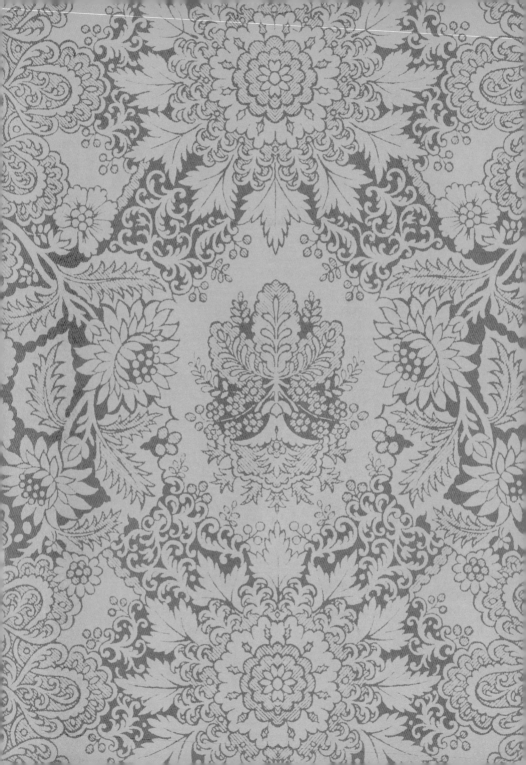

ALSO BY

NINA GARCIA

AND ILLUSTRATED BY

RUBEN TOLEDO

THE LITTLE BLACK BOOK OF STYLE

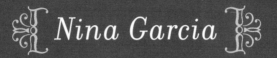

Nina Garcia

ILLUSTRATIONS BY

RUBEN TOLEDO

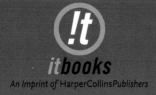

itbooks

An Imprint of HarperCollinsPublishers

The ONE HUNDRED

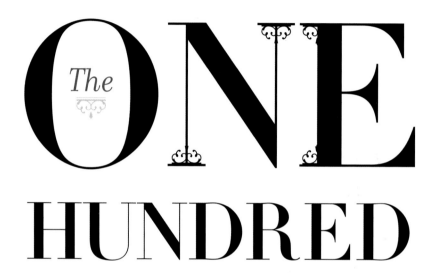

A GUIDE TO
THE PIECES EVERY STYLISH
WOMAN MUST OWN

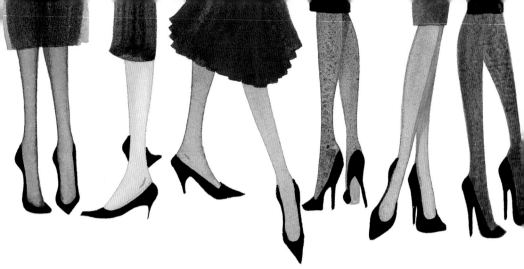

First It Books paperback published 2010.

Book design by Shubhani Sarkar

Library of Congress Cataloging-in-Publication Data

Garcia, Nina.
  The one hundred: a guide to the pieces every stylish woman must own/
Nina Garcia; illustrations by Ruben Toledo.—1st ed.
    p. cm.
  ISBN 978-0-06-166461-8
1. Dress accessories. 2. Fashion. 3. Women's clothing. I. Title. II. Title:
One hundred. III. Title: 100.
  TT649.8.G27 2008
  687.082—dc22   2008018585

  ISBN 978-0-06-166463-2 (pbk.)

10   11   12   13   14   ID/SCP   10   9   8   7   6   5   4   3   2

Raindrops on roses and whiskers on kittens
Bright copper kettles and warm woolen mittens
Brown paper packages tied up with strings
These are a few of my favorite things. . .

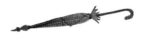

Contents

Author's Note   xiii

A

1. A-Line Dress   2
2. Animal Print   5
3. Ankle Bootie   8
4. Aviators   10

B

5. Ballet Flat   16
6. Bangles   18
7. Belts   23
8. Bikini   25
9. BlackBerry   28
10. Black Opaque Tights   31
11. Blazer   34
12. Boyfriend Cardigan   36
13. Brooch   38

C

14. Cable-Knit Sweater   42
15. Caftan   44
16. Camel Coat   46
17. Cape   48
18. Cashmere Sweater   50
19. Charm Bracelet   52
20. Clutch   56
21. Cocktail Ring   61
22. Converse   64
23. Cosmetics Bag   66
24. Cowboy Boots   70
25. Cuff   73

D E F

26.	Denim Jacket	78
27.	Diamond Studs	80
28.	Driving Shoe	82
29.	Espadrilles	84
30.	Evening Gown	87
31.	Exotic Skin Bag	89
32.	Fishnets	91
33.	Frye Harness Boot	94
34.	Fur	96

G H I

35.	Gentlemen's Hat	102
36.	Gloves	105
37.	Havaianas	108
38.	Hobo Bag	111
39.	Hoop Earrings	112
40.	Investment Bag	114
41.	iPod	120

J K L

42.	Jeans	125
43.	Jewelry Pouches	129
44.	Khakis	130
45.	Knee Boots	131
46.	Leather Pants	134
47.	Lingerie	136
48.	Little Black Dress	139
49.	Little White Dress	144
50.	L.L.Bean Tote	146
51.	Luggage	149

M
N
O

52. Mad Money   154
53. Man's White Shirt   155
54. Mary Janes   158
55. Minnetonka Moccasin   162
56. Missoni Knit   165
57. Monogrammed Stationery   168
58. Motorcycle Jacket   170
59. Nail Polish   174
60. Old Concert T-Shirt   176
61. One-Piece Swimsuit   178

P
Q
R

62. Pajamas   182
63. Peacoat   184
64. Pearl Necklace   187
65. Pencil Skirt   188
66. Perfume   191
67. Plain White Tee   194
68. Polo Shirt   197
69. Pucci   201
70. Push-Up Bra   203
71. Quality Champagne   205
72. Red Lipstick   207
73. Robe   210

S

74. Safari Jacket   214
75. Sandals   216
76. Sarong   219
77. Signet Ring   221

S

78.	Silk Scarf	223
79.	Slippers	226
80.	Spanx	229
81.	Statement Necklace	230
82.	Stilettos	233
83.	Striped Sailor Shirt	235
84.	Suit	237
85.	Sunhat	240

T U V

86.	Trench	244
87.	Turquoise and Coral Jewelry	247
88.	Tuxedo Jacket	249
89.	Umbrella	252
90.	Underwear	254
91.	Valid Passport	257
92.	Vans	258
93.	Vintage	260

W Y Z

94.	Watch	264
95.	Wayfarers	266
96.	Wellington Boot	268
97.	Wide-Leg Trousers	270
98.	Wrap Dress	273
99.	Yoga Gear	275
100.	Zippered Hoodie	277

Parting Words . . .	281
Acknowledgments	283

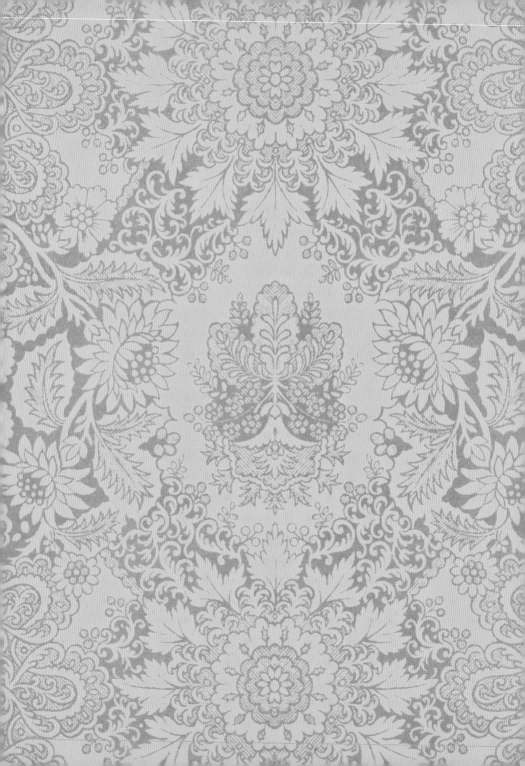

Author's Note

I F YOU WALKED INTO MY CLOSET at this very moment, what would you see? Racks of shoes and stacks of bags. Piles of white Hanes T-shirts and black cashmere sweaters. A row of black dresses and a shelf devoted entirely to denim. And over it all, you would see a big, ugly canvas tarp. I am in the throes of an apartment remodel, which was supposed to be finished in November. Of 2006. It is now March. Of 2008. My husband, my son, and I have been holing up at a place a few blocks away. Every once in a while I'll run back to the apartment, step over the dust and debris, make my way to my old closet, lift off the canvas tarp, and snatch an item or two.

Over the months, I must have run back about a hundred times. And soon I realized that I had the answer to the questions that women keep asking me: What are the essentials? What are the "must-haves"? Well, for me, the must-haves are the items I run back to my apartment for, the items I have stepped over dust and debris for—they are the items I *simply cannot imagine* living without.

And why?

Because these items have been there with me season after season. They have been with me through thick and thin. When trends begin to fade away, these are the items I can always turn to with confidence. Each has alternately comforted me when I'm down after a bad, grueling day, and each in turn has boosted my confidence to greater heights when I'm feeling great after a good, fulfilling day. Each has its place in my heart. Each represents the yin and yang of my personal style.

Simply put, these items make me feel *classic*. And there is no substitute for feeling this way. Ever.

In my years as a fashion director, I have watched many fads come and go, but I have also observed how certain items are always a part of the rotation. Some may sit out for a year or two (perhaps even more), but they always come back. The color may change, the fabric may change, the designer or brand may change, but in essence, the items in this book have always been the backbone of fashion, and, with a bit of self-editing, each has been one of my style touchstones.

But self-editing is key.

It is important for everyone who reads this book to know that I have adapted and edited each item on this list to suit *my* style, *my* body, *my* personality. I should hope you will do the same. This book is designed to be a sort of shopping list of or guide to the items I feel every woman should have, but it is certainly not the end-all be-all. There is no *ultimate* list, as it would go against the very nature of fashion and style, and the frenetic rebelliousness inherent in a truly stylish woman walking down the street wearing that perfectly unexpected mix of color and fabric. Style is dangerously unpredictable. What I have done here is to give every woman a framework to think and ponder. This list is a guide, a barometer of industry items that have withstood time and seasons, fads and trends.

So when you take this list of One Hundred, I hope that you remember the tenet I set down in my first book, *The Little Black Book of Style:* **Style is a deeply personal expression of who you are, and**

every time you dress, you are asserting a part of yourself. Remember this as you read this book, as you think of what your own One Hundred will be.

Thus, if you are not altering each or some of the items on this list to suit *your* personal style, you are not playing the style game correctly or for your benefit. You see, no matter how you picture yourself in your own personal fashion spread of the imagination or what your personal style may be, we all rely on the few fashion items that really are our style pillars. The following items are mine. And I bet many of these could be (should be!) yours as well.

So, with that said, I give you my essential One Hundred. From the A-Line Dress to Converse sneaks, from the Cocktail Ring to the Little Black Dress, these are the pieces that have stood the test of time. Both with myself, as well as within the fashion industry I have devoted my professional life connecting to, loving, being inspired by. These items are as personal as any woman gets—reading this book is, after all, like walking you into my closet. And, as any woman knows, opening up your closet can be like telling your best friend your untold secrets: Her reaction may surprise you. With any luck, my One Hundred will do just that.

Shoppers, take your marks,

Nina

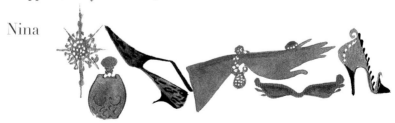

P.S. She who dies with the most stilettos wins.

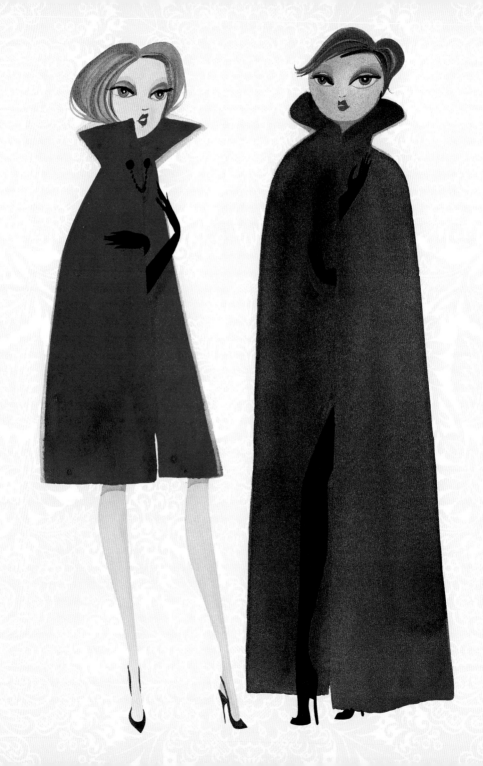

. . . When the dog bites
When the bee stings
When I'm feeling sad
I simply remember my favorite things
And then I don't feel so bad.

STILL FROM "MY FAVORITE THINGS,"

RODGERS AND HAMMERSTEIN,

FROM *THE SOUND OF MUSIC*

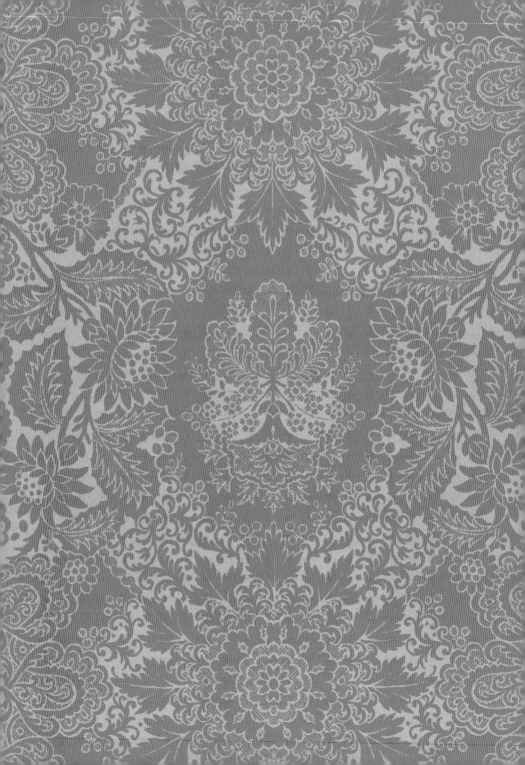

The ONE
HUNDRED

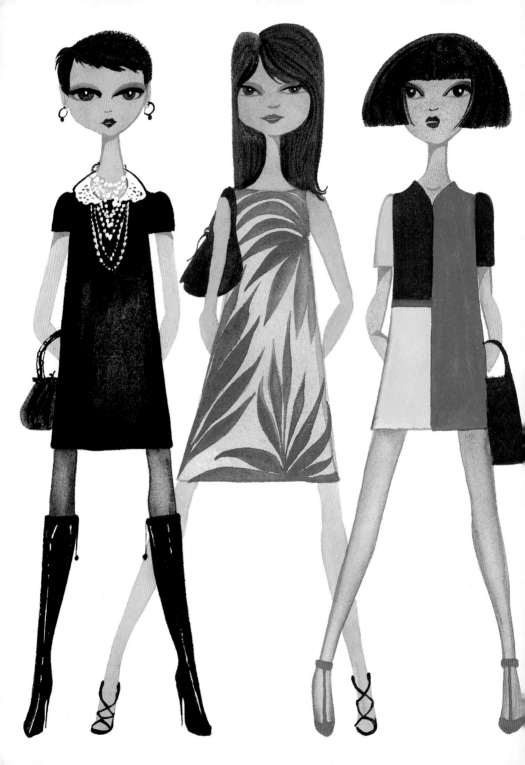

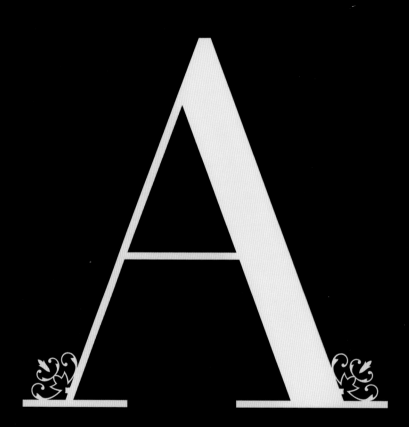

1.
A-Line Dress

TRUE A-LINE is narrower on the top and flares out gently toward the bottom, resembling the letter A, thus the name. Here's the deal with the A-line dress: It *will* work for you on your *best* day. It *will* work for you on your *worst* day. It *will* work when you don't know what to wear, for all occasions, and in all kinds of weather. And no matter what, it *will* flatter your figure. That is really a lot for a fashion item to give you. Yet, it demands so little in return, just a few bold accessories, a great pair of shoes, and maybe a pair of tights, depending on the time of year. But that's it. It is a no-fuss dress and perhaps that is why it was the must-have dress of the '60s, when fun and free-spiritedness was favored over the formality and structure of the prior decade.

Every '60s "It" girl had an arsenal of these dresses in her closet—Twiggy, Penelope Tree, Edie Sedgwick, Mary Quant, Jean Shrimpton. These were the Kate Mosses of the day. If you do a Google image search of these women, a picture of them in an A-line will always come up on the first page. They are often wearing a bold print or a bright-colored A-line with boots or flats. Their accessories are always amazing. This became the unofficial uniform of the 1960s, and the reason this dress should still be in every girl's closet today is because it is so damn flattering. Eat, ladies, for we always have the A-line.

With a good A-line, the fabric flows over perceived flaws or imperfections. No matter the day, the season, or the year, the A-line dress will always make you look and feel fashionable, fabulous, and perfectly capable of keeping up with Twiggy and her crew.

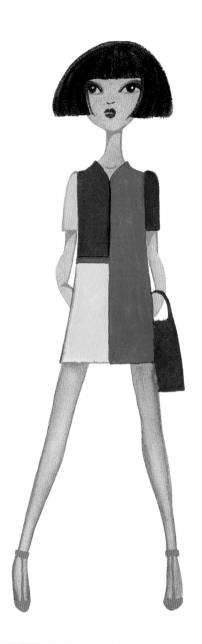

GET IN LINE

- It is advisable to always have a black A-line in your repertoire as a "just in case" dress. As in: just in case you are invited to a dinner party or out on an impromptu date and only have five minutes to get ready.
- The dress is perfect to wear in the summer with Sandals (#75) or in the winter with Knee Boots (#45). A dress for all seasons, indeed.
- For a great contrast, wear a white A-line with your Black Opaque Tights (see #10). The look is always youthful and playful.
- If you want to really be daring, wear a bright-colored A-line with a bright-colored tight, like a true '60s mod girl.

fashion
101

TYPE A

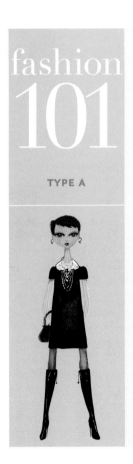

Christian Dior created the A-line dress in 1955, a style he had adapted from Cristobal Balenciaga's more extreme trapeze dress. Dior cut off a lot of the excess fabric from the sides and created a silhouette that was more streamlined, but still fit loose on the body. In the 1950s, women were used to wearing tighter, waist-accentuating designs, and the A-line was anything but. At first, women rejected this new style of dress, its shape, its informality. They hadn't been dieting for nothing! But in the '60s, when girls were eager to be freed from the constraints of all of those waist-conscious designs, the A-line started to take off. When women like Twiggy and Jackie O became fans, it was all the celebrity endorsement the A-line needed to secure its reputation in the annals of fashion history.

The fashionable woman wears clothes.
The clothes don't wear her.

MARY QUANT

2.
Animal Print

THE TRULY FASHIONABLE are always daring and never dull. They are willing to run with the leopards, the cheetahs, the zebras. And in our urban-inspired lives in cities like New York, Miami, Chicago, LA, more than ever our way of life resembles the jungles and savannahs of Africa or South America. We're wild. Child. And sometimes we need to show it a little.

An animal-print accessory is an opportunity to be a little bold. It allows you to throw in that slight element of danger on an otherwise safe outfit and let the world know there is more to you than meets the eye. A full-on leopard-print dress, on the other hand, sends the clear message that you are no wallflower, you are a force to be reckoned with. But there is a fine line between looking chic and looking tawdry when wearing an animal print. Keep this in mind when you're ready to let the world see a piece of your primal side.

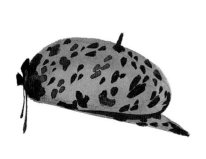 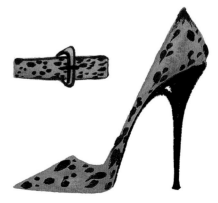

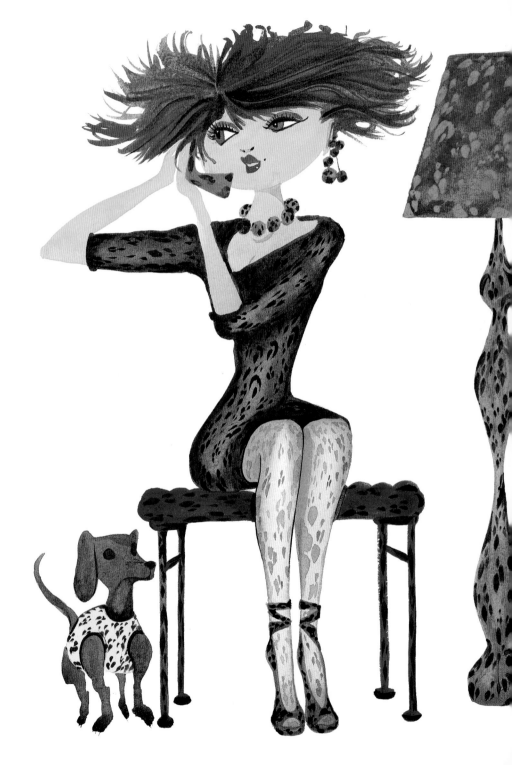

WELCOME TO THE JUNGLE

To keep your cool, remember:

- Buying a print with pedigree (think Dolce & Gabbana or YSL) is the best way to avoid the garish look that is sometimes associated with animal prints. There are items that you can save money on. This should not be one of them.
- Wear only one piece of animal print at a time. Any more than that and you will look like fashion roadkill.
- Keep everything else simple, even severe. Pair the print with neutral colors (black, white, camel, khaki). Keep everything else classic and the print will carry itself.
- When shopping, remember that on a good animal print, the colors are muted (never pink or blue or yellow!). Less is more, but none gets you nowhere!

Why make everything black, black, black?
Fashion should be fun and put a woman in the
spotlight with a little bit of danger, you know?

ROBERTO CAVALLI

3.

Ankle Bootie

THE ANKLE BOOT was originally intended to be hidden beneath classic trousers. Ankle boots with skirts? Unthinkable! But when the bootie got into the hands of designers like Christian Louboutin and Miuccia Prada, it was transformed. Just like that. I remember in the '80s when designers first put the bootie on the runways with skirts and dresses. It caused a bit of a frenzy, and everyone wondered why we had been hiding these shoes under our pants for so long. Women began wearing them with everything *but* classic trousers: dresses, drainpipes, and the very intrepid (and genetically blessed) wore them with shorts. And now, who can think of a world where ankle boots are not meant to come out and play? It seems as though they never had any other purpose than to make us look and feel a little punk when sporting them with skirts or skinny jeans.

One of these days
these boots are gonna walk all over you.

NANCY SINATRA

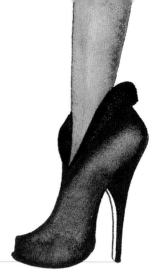

BOOTIE CALL

- When wearing with pants, keep the colors the same. Black skinny pants tucked into black booties will elongate the leg and make you feel fabulous.
- When wearing with miniskirts, try them with Black Opaque Tights (#10) to keep your line going and going and going. Unless you have fabulous legs, illusion is our master craft.
- Make sure the bootie does not cut off straight at the ankle like a traditional bootie—these boots are made to be worn under pants and will chop off the leg and make it look stumpy.
- It is a great alternative to the pump—always consider it if the pump seems too safe.
- The bootie is a classic way to mix the masculine with the feminine, so don't be afraid to flaunt a little femininity when you have this more masculine shoe on. One must mix it to risk it. . . .

4.
Aviators

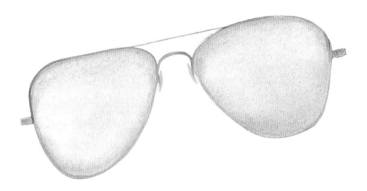

T HINK KATE HUDSON in *Almost Famous*, Tom Cruise in *Top Gun*, Brad Pitt in *Fight Club*, Leonardo DiCaprio in *The Aviator*. The beauty of Aviator sunglasses is that they look perfect on the groupie from the '70s (Penny Lane), the fighter pilot from the '80s (Maverick), the lunatic from the '90s (Tyler Durden), and of course an aviator from the '30s (Howard Hughes). They are an eternally and universally fashionable shade that instantly brings out that cool factor. Wear them with your oldest jeans or with your newest tailored YSL jacket and look equally up-to-the-minute.

- The classic Aviator is the Ray-Ban, but almost every designer at almost every price point makes a good version. Keep it as close to the original design as possible. Michael Kors and Ralph Lauren do it very well.
- Stay away from too much shine. Nothing takes away the cool factor quite like reflective lenses or shiny rims. The rims should be in a matte tone of silver or gold.
- Look for vintage versions. The more history they have, the better, the classier, the more you smolder when wearing them.

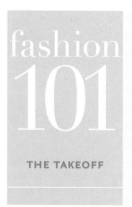

fashion
101

THE TAKEOFF

In 1936, the U.S. government commissioned Ray-Ban to design sunglasses for Air Force pilots. The pilots wanted something that would provide the protection of their aviation goggles without the bulk. Ray-Ban came up with the Aviator design, which was an immediate hit. After more than seventy years, the sunglasses have maintained their popularity, and the model that aviators wore in 1936 is the same model that fashionistas and celebrities still wear today.

FAMOUS FANS

Madonna	Steve McQueen	Angelina Jolie
Kate Hudson	Jim Morrison	Jack Nicholson
Marlon Brando	Steven Tyler	Lauren Hutton

Any of you boys seen an aircraft carrier around here?

MAVERICK, *TOP GUN*

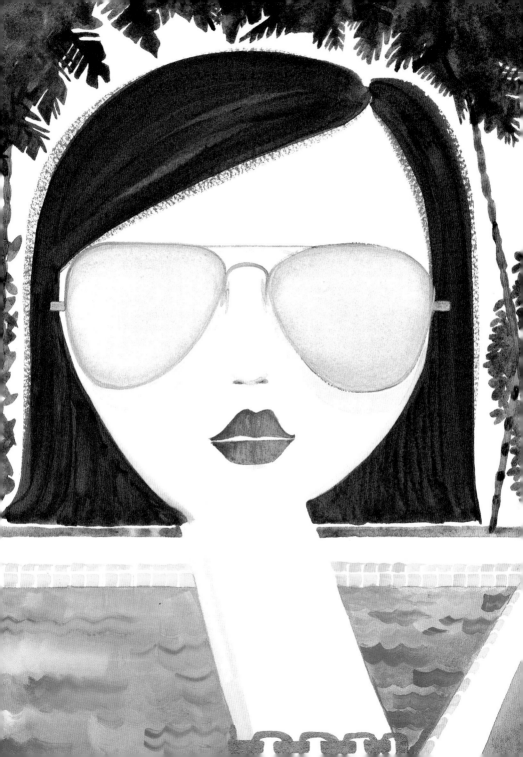

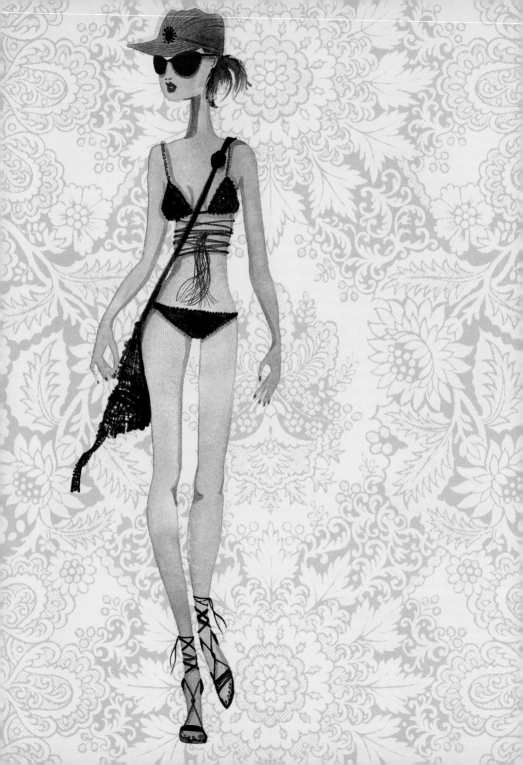

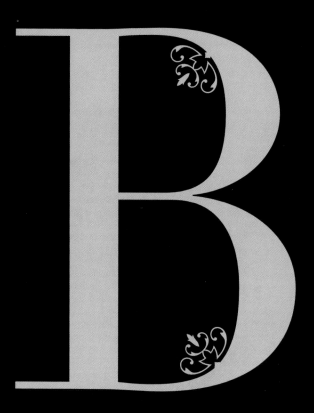

5.
Ballet Flat

THOUGH IT WILL NEVER HAVE the transformative power of the high heel, a ballet flat is chic and timeless in its own right. It is simple and elegant, and it remains one of the few flat shoes that the fashion world has adopted and adored. And it's comfortable! From sex vixen Brigitte Bardot, to the impeccable Audrey Hepburn, to every Hollywood starlet in between, the ballet flat has always had its fair share of famous fans, and it has become the go-to shoe for those few times when a heel is out of the question. But when a gal is hitting the town, it is best to throw the flats into your bag, because every stylish girl knows that when the sun goes down, the heel goes up, and as gravity teaches, all things must come down. And the classic ballet flat will be waiting for you when it does.

The only sin is mediocrity.

MARTHA GRAHAM

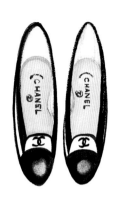

- Repetto is the classic, French original, but many companies make a good version. For a high-end pair try Chanel (with the black toe cap) or Lanvin. For a more inexpensive option, check Gap, J.Crew, Tory Burch, H&M.
- Though you cannot go wrong with a black pair, consider something fun, too. Look for a bright color, a skin, or a bold pattern.

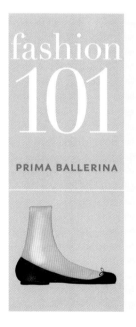

fashion 101

PRIMA BALLERINA

Before she was an actress, a sex kitten, and a fashion icon, Brigitte Bardot was a trained ballet dancer. She was also a loyal and devoted fan of Repetto pointe shoes. When Bardot signed on to be in Roger Vadim's 1956 film, *And God Created Woman*, she asked Rose Repetto to make her a pair of flats to wear during that now legendary mambo scene. Mme Repetto, working out of her tiny walk-up shop on Rue de la Paix, created a pair of crimson flats for Bardot, which the actress instantly adored. When the film debuted, Bardot and the ballet flats became overnight sensations. Then, a year later, when Hepburn donned her own pair for her dancing scene in *Funny Face*, the shoes once again flew from the silver screen to the streets. Now, fifty years later, the same ballet flats that Bardot and Hepburn adored are as desirable as ever.

6.
Bangles

⸺∾⸺

THE YOUNG, COOL MODELS wear fun, colorful, plastic versions with their T-shirts and Converse. Actresses often choose to wear a pile of thin gold ones as their armor on the red carpet. And the "It" girls go for funky ethnic styles from India and Africa. Bangles are a style staple that let a girl play around. They are available in an array of precious and nonprecious materials. You can find them in Saks or on the street. They can be extremely plain or intricately decorated. Bright and bold, or more classic and traditional. It all depends on your style. Try out different versions. Mix the wood with the silver. See what works for you. Your bangles are your bells, announcing your stylish arrival.

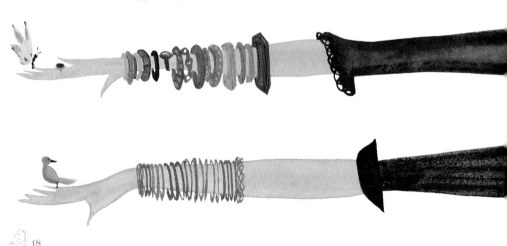

- Rare vintage Bakelite bangles: Bakelite is a very rare, very beautiful material produced in the 1920s and '30s, but is no longer manufactured. Check out Mark Davis or scour the vintage shops.
- Hermès enamel bangles: The iconic bangle, which comes in a variety of designs. Great when stacked together or mixed with other colors.
- Alexis Bittar: Designer who makes beautiful Lucite bangles.

ARM CANDY

- For the bold, wear big designs from wrist to elbow, as Nancy Cunard famously did. (Google: *Nancy Cunard in bangles*. You won't be disappointed.)
- For glamour, wear an armload of thin eighteen-carat gold bracelets à la Carolina Herrera, who is known for wearing at least ten at a time. You should stick to no less than six. Mix inexpensive and real if you'd like. It's good to go vintage here.
- For fun, look for odd-colored Bakelite from the flea market or cheap Indian bangles.
- For a little glitz, thin bangles of small pavé diamonds add fun and sparkle.

fashion
101

BAKELITE BANGLES

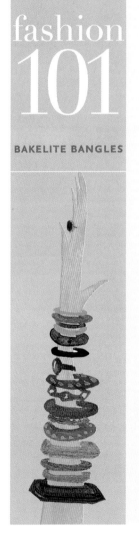

Bakelite is a very rare material that is no longer made. It was the precursor to plastic, was almost indestructible, could easily imitate other materials (ivory, tortoiseshell, coral), and could be dyed almost any color. It was used from the 1920s through the 1950s to make everything from telephone handsets to radios to buttons to costume jewelry. Bakelite jewelry pieces became popular in the '20s and gained momentum as the Depression deepened and buying expensive jewelry was out of the question. Women wore colorful Bakelite bangles to add color and a bit of fun to an otherwise drab period. Icons like Diana Vreeland and Elsa Schiaparelli were fans of the bangles and helped to contribute to the popularity of the jewelry. When World War II began, production of Bakelite ground to a halt, since factories were used to make war materials only. By the time the war was over, cheaper plastics had been developed and very little of the material was produced. The golden age of Bakelite had ended. Today, costume jewelry made out of Bakelite is highly collectible.

The most sought-after colors include:

- **BUTTERSCOTCH,** a golden yellow, which was produced only during the '30s.
- **"END OF DAY,"** a blend of three or more contrasting colors, which were put together in the factory at the end of the day with all of the leftover materials.
- **STARDUST,** transparent with specks of gold, which disappeared after the 1930s.

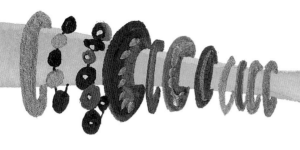

It is the unseen, unforgettable,
ultimate accessory of fashion
that heralds your arrival
and prolongs your departure.

COCO CHANEL

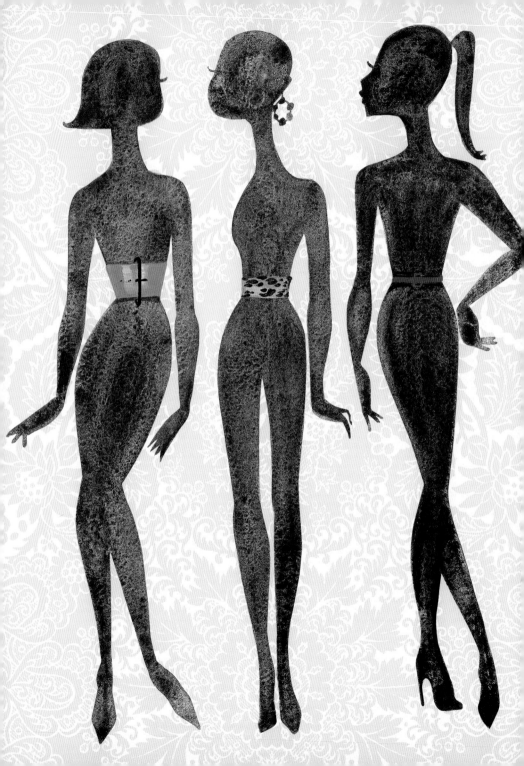

7

Belts

⊗∞⊗

A N OFTEN OVERLOOKED and underappreciated accessory (shoes and bags get all the attention). Yet, a great
belt can make you look slimmer, pulled together, ac-
centuate curves, and add bling to an otherwise bland
outfit. A thick black belt on a black dress instantly
narrows the waist and highlights your curves. A hip belt on top of a
tunic will draw the eye down. A skinny belt on a low-slung trouser
makes you look polished. But the belt is not just about the silhouette.
Think of your belts as pieces of jewelry. Look for unique designs,
styles, fabrics, and big buckles. Try out corset belts, hip belts, ethnic
styles, red crocodile, green python, zebra print, etc., etc. These are
the kinds of belts that you can add to a white dress, a black dress, or
jeans and a T-shirt—and in seconds the look is transformed.

THE INSIDE TRACK: **MY FAVORITES**

- LAI (Luxury Accessories International): If you want a really
skinny belt, LAI is the place.
- Lana Marks: The best crocodile belts.
- Streets Ahead: The source for studded rocker belts.
- Linea Pelle: Italian craftsmanship at its finest.

- Some seasons it is not a "belt year," and designers are not making many. But you are almost certain to find a good belt at these top-end designers, who always carry really good belts: **Dolce & Gabbana, Gucci, Lanvin, Ralph Lauren, Azzedine Alaia.**

BUCKLE UP

- A wide belt around the slimmest part of your waist creates an instant hourglass. Cinch it!
- If the belt is big and/or bold, keep the jewelry simple. Let the belt be the focal point.
- A skinny belt works best with a low-slung or high-waisted trouser.
- A belt is a great way to get a piece of a designer collection without spending a fortune. Most designers will have a signature belt each season, and if you can get your hands on it, you'll be able to achieve the look without splurging for the entire outfit.

A waist is a terrible thing to waste.

ANONYMOUS

8.
Bikini

⊂∞∞⊃

THE KEY TO WEARING A BIKINI is confidence, confidence, confidence. The girls that rock a bikini best do not necessarily have the most perfect bodies. But they do have the perfect outlook. They realize that when you are lucky enough to be by a pool or an ocean, obsessing about your body is the least stylish thing in the world.

That being said, when shopping for the bikini, always keep in mind that the mirrors in the dressing rooms are always wrong and the lighting is always off. It is an evil situation and should only be entered into with a best friend or sister so that you can remind each other that with tans and drinks in your hands, you'll look amazing.

BATHING BEAUTIES

1. Stick to sophisticated, solid colors (black, navy, gray, chocolate brown, white). Leave the patterns and crazy colors to the fifteen-year-olds.
2. Smaller is more flattering. It should not be too big, especially on the bottom, as it will bunch up, perhaps sag, and look terrible. Mix-and-match bottoms and don't play by any rules. Bikini Time is Bikini Time. Enough said.

There are a number of designers who really know how to make a great swimsuit. What sets them apart is the quality of the Lycra (it is thick and durable), the saturated colors, and the fine hardware. Look for these characteristics when bathing-suit shopping. Here are my favorites:

· Onda de Mar
· Rosa Chá
· Eres
· Ralph Lauren
· Tomas Maier

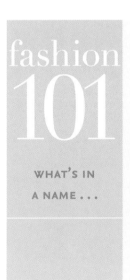

fashion
101

WHAT'S IN

A NAME . . .

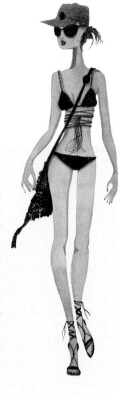

The bikini got its name because it debuted during the same time that nuclear testing began on Bikini Atoll. The French inventors, engineer Louis Réard and fashion designer Jacques Heim, dubbed their creation the bikini, as they thought it might receive an explosive reaction. Smart men. They were right.

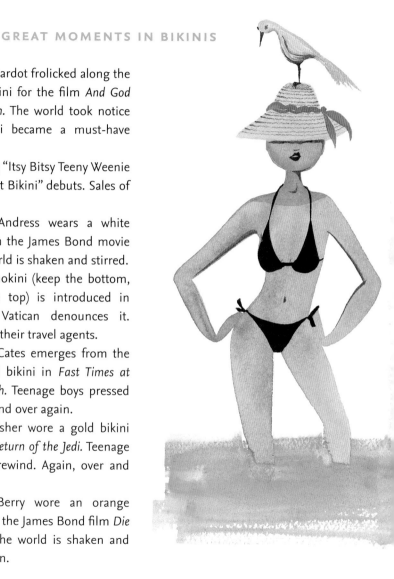

- 1957: Brigitte Bardot frolicked along the beach in a bikini for the film *And God Created Woman*. The world took notice and the bikini became a must-have item.
- 1960: The song "Itsy Bitsy Teeny Weenie Yellow Polkadot Bikini" debuts. Sales of the bikini soar.
- 1962: Ursula Andress wears a white belted bikini in the James Bond movie *Dr. No*. The world is shaken and stirred.
- 1964: The monokini (keep the bottom, take away the top) is introduced in Europe. The Vatican denounces it. Americans call their travel agents.
- 1982: Phoebe Cates emerges from the water in a red bikini in *Fast Times at Ridgemont High*. Teenage boys pressed rewind. Over and over again.
- 1983: Carrie Fisher wore a gold bikini in *Star Wars: Return of the Jedi*. Teenage boys pressed rewind. Again, over and over.
- 2002: Halle Berry wore an orange belted bikini in the James Bond film *Die Another Day*. The world is shaken and stirred . . . again.

9.
BlackBerry

LSO KNOWN AS the "CrackBerry" for its strongly addictive qualities. It is the modern girl's weapon. It allows her to bid on eBay when walking down the street, map out her shopping route for maximum productivity, and sneak out of work and still get her messages as she peruses the sales racks. It also lets her check out Perez Hilton and Fashion Week Daily while waiting for lunch dates to arrive, planes to board, shops to open, etc.

It is an essential accessory for keeping in touch with loved ones and keeping oneself wired to the world at large.

FUN FACT

The term *CrackBerry* became so popular that in November 2006 it made Webster's New World College Dictionary as the New Word of the Year.

MY FAVORITE SITES

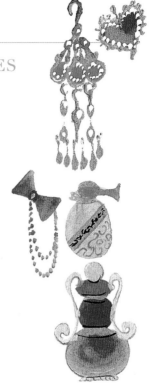

FOR CELEB UPDATES

- pinkisthenewblog.com
- perezhilton.com
- jossip.com

FOR FASHION UPDATES

- fashionweekdaily.com
- style.com
- fashionista.com
- fabsugar.com
- bagsnob.com

FOR SHOPPING DEALS (AND SPLURGES)

- bluefly.com
- net-a-porter.com
- couturelab.com

Lo! Men have become the tools of their tools.

HENRY DAVID THOREAU

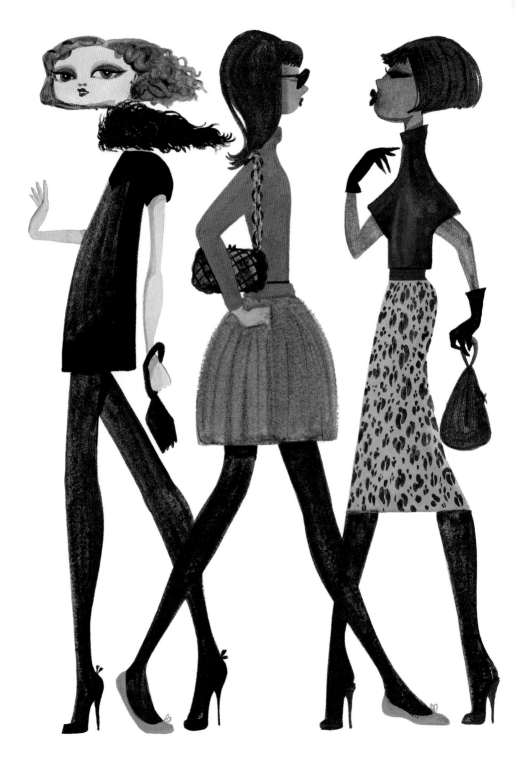

10.
Black Opaque Tights

I N THE 1960S, when short skirts and minidresses and Edie Sedgwick walked the streets, black opaque tights became a staple. Edie, the original black opaque tight girl, would wear them with everything: her shift dresses, her extra-long T-shirts, her signature leotards. She showed the world how a simple bit of legwear constituted consummate hipness. And the rest of the mod girls would wear these tights with the shortest of skirts and still manage to look stylish instead of scandalous. The black opaque leg may have started in the '60s, but it continues to march its way into every decade, not just for the edge it can bring to an outfit, but also because it can miraculously make the leg look sleeker, longer, and slimmer.

FUN FACT

Denier is the measure of density for tights and pantyhose. Tne higher the denier, the more opaque the hose. The sheerest denier is 5; the most opaque is 80.

Tip: Try a pair of ribbed tights for an extra-lengthening effect.

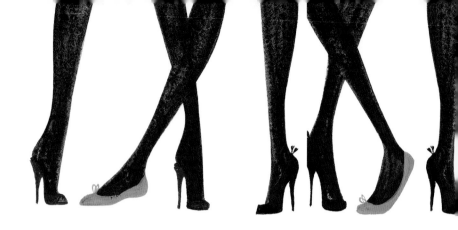

A LEG UP

- Wear black tights with black suede boots or a black heel so the eye sees one long, sleek line.
- Use contrast. A black leg under a bright white dress makes the look pop.
- If a skirt is questionably short, a black leg will make it fashionably short.
- Do not buy cheap. You don't want to see any skin through the tight, and you don't want to have them show as uneven or splotchy—this ruins the whole look!
- From time to time, you may see a girl wearing her black opaque tights as pants. They are, in fact, not.

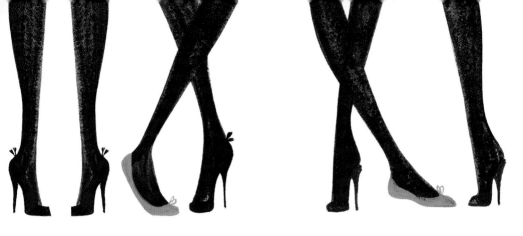

CLOSET OBSESSION: **WOLFORD**

The reason I will spend $50–80 on a pair of Wolfords is because they are the black tights with the most opaque/matte combination (no skin showing through, no splotchiness, no shine), which is key when wearing black tights. They use a unique knitting system of blending Lycra into the knit, which ensures maximum opaqueness, comfort, and durability, all of which make it worth the extra cost.

Fogal is another brand that must be mentioned. It is rumored to have been Jackie O's brand of choice and is still a favorite among the fashion circles.

MY FAVORITE PAIRS

· Wolford Velvet de Luxe 66: Opaque, matte, with just the tiniest bit of sheer.
· Wolford Matte Opaque 80: Ballet dancers' black. No sheer at all.

11.
Blazer

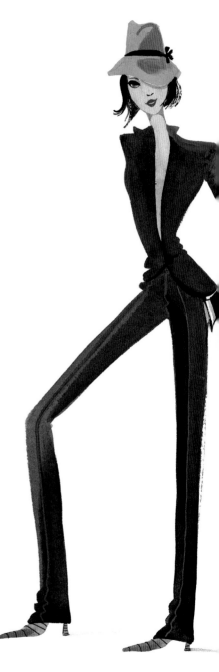

THE JACKET that women blatantly stole from the boys and then wore it better, as is so often the case. Women wear it with sleek white pants or on top of little black dresses; we wear it with skinny black jeans or khakis (Google *Balenciaga Fall 2007*). Girls most often wear it with heels instead of the standard prep-school penny loafers. The beauty of the blazer is that it does a tango between the masculine and the feminine, the formal and the casual, the preppy and the trendy, the smart and the sexy. You can't quite pin it down, and therein lies its charm. A chic untraditional way to buy a blazer is to buy it unconstructed or oversized (Google *Ann Demeulemeester*) or shrunken (Brooks Brothers boys' department) for a dramatic and fashionable look.

TAILOR MADE

- THE BUTTONS: Make sure they are working buttons with real buttonholes. It is a sign of a quality blazer.
- THE SLEEVES: Should fall at the heel of your hand for a traditional and timeless look. If you want to take it in a trendier direction, you can go about an inch longer than the traditional sleeve length, or choose a three-quarter length.
- THE SHOULDERS: Should be straight and crisp. The seam where the arm and body meet should be at the outer edge of your shoulder.
- THE FRONT: Should lie smooth when buttoned. Even if you never button your blazer, make sure you button it at the tailor so you can make sure there are no bumps or bulges. (In fact, check for bumps and bulges everywhere else, too.)
- THE LENGTH: It is all a matter of preference. The classic blazer will fall at your hip, but it can be longer or cropped, depending on your personal style.
- FINAL TEST: While you are still at the tailor, lift your hands above your head, reach out in front, etc. The blazer should move with you, never pulling or bunching.

12.
Boyfriend Cardigan

GO AHEAD, STEAL IT. Or at least borrow it for a very, very long time. Take his cardigan. Dads, grandpas, brothers, friends, and roommates are all fair game, too. The boyfriend cardigan had a high-fashion moment when Marc Jacobs did grunge and the models appeared on the runway with skirts, combat boots, and oversized cardigans. But the boyfriend cardigan had been around long before grunge and will remain long after. Perhaps because anything that looks like it was stolen out of your boyfriend's closet will never go out of style.

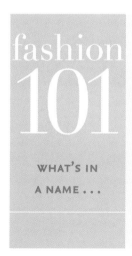

fashion
101

WHAT'S IN

A NAME . . .

The cardigan got its origin and its name in 1854, when the seventh Earl of Cardigan needed an extra layer of warmth under his uniform during the Crimean War. He got it—he got warm. We ladies got something to stylistically play with forever.

COZY UP

- The best version to look for has four buttons, with two pockets at the front.
- There are great resources to be tapped in the men's sections of Neiman Marcus, Bergdorf Goodman, Gap, Target, H&M.
- Wear it over a very fine tank top or T-shirt and then belt it.
- Experiment. Try wearing it over a feminine dress with boots.
- Use it as a jacket in the fall or spring to look casual and low-key.

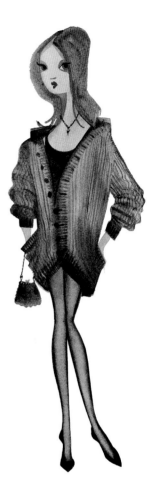

Dressing is a way of life.

YVES SAINT LAURENT

13.
Brooch

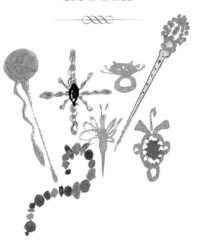

THE UNINITIATED associate the brooch with grand-mothers and great-aunts and think it is only to be worn on the neckline of dresses. But the fashionable are aware that it is capable of so much more. It is an accessory that allows you to show off your creative side. Find ironic designs and large, interesting pieces. Put them in your hair, on your hats, on unexpected places on your clothing. Follow the lead of women like Sharon Stone, who tied back her husband's white shirt with a dragonfly pin and stepped out on the red carpet in 1998. Or Charlize Theron, who ingeniously placed a brooch on each strap of her amber Vera Wang dress for the 2000 Oscars. A few years later, she placed two diamond flower brooches in her perfectly coiffed hair. Google these images, and then go scour the vintage shops and your grandma's jewelry box to find brooches you can play around with.

GREAT MOMENTS IN BROOCHES

- 1975: In the film *Grey Gardens*, Edith Bouvier Beale famously finished off every outfit with a four-inch brooch. It is iconic enough to have its own Web site, thegreygardensbrooch.com.
- 1994: Madeleine Albright was meeting with an Iraqi foreign minister who had previously called her a snake. She wore a snake brooch.
- 1998: Eva Peron's diamond-and-sapphire brooch of the flag of Argentina sold at auction for $992,500 to an anonymous American bidder (rumored to be Madonna).

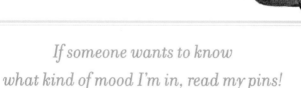

*If someone wants to know
what kind of mood I'm in, read my pins!*

MADELEINE ALBRIGHT

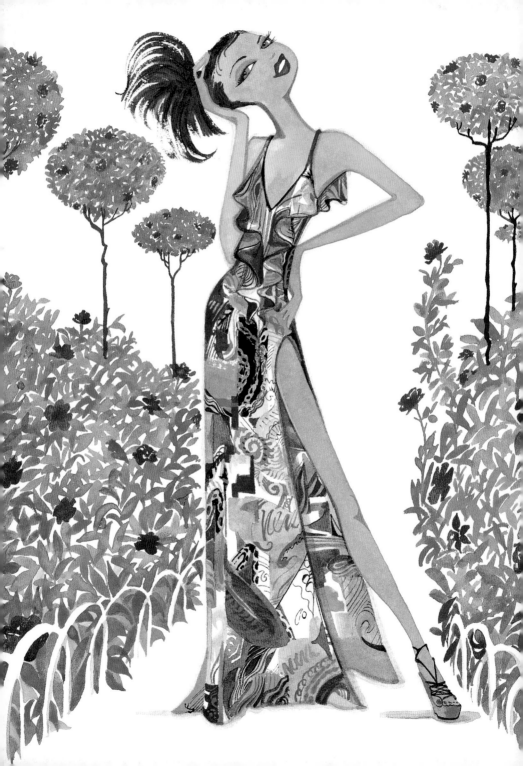

14.

Cable-Knit Sweater

THE CABLE-KNIT SWEATER, also known as the fisherman's sweater, has its roots in Ireland, but has since become a New England tradition (think Ali McGraw in *Love Story*). The cable-knit will always be seen as classically preppy (think Ralph Lauren), but it can also be runway-worthy (look at how Michael Kors and Chloé updated the classic). There is a version of the cable-knit for every aspect of one's personal style. Find your match, and you will have a go-to garment for the rest of your life. Whichever version you go with, it will remain the kind of wardrobe staple that allows you to be cozy and casual, yet unbelievably stylish at the same time. The cable-knit sweater sends that message of casual indifference ("Oh, just something I threw on"). And yet it also sends a message of supreme style (" . . . but I knew what I was doing").

And one must always send a message.

I always wear my sweater back-to-front;
it is so much more flattering.

DIANA VREELAND

- Weekend Casual: Find an oversized oatmeal version with skinny jeans tucked into harness boots.
- Supremely Sophisticated: Wear a white fitted cable-knit with white pants and a camel coat thrown on top.
- Thoroughly Modern: Seek out a cashmere dress version and pair it with a belt and a boot.
- Prep School Chic: Stay true to its roots, and wear a J.Crew version with chinos and moccasins.

CABLE BOX

- A perfect white version can be an ideal travel sweater, since it is likely to go with almost everything in your suitcase.
- Wear a skinny pant or cigarette pant to even out the volume on top. Any volume on both the bottom *and* top is going to make you look huge. Balance is key.
- This is a fun item to buy in the men's department (again!), but be extra-careful of fit (in case you haven't noticed, boys aren't exactly built like us).
- Chloé makes the ultimate fashion version, if you want to invest. Keep everything else neat and simple—the hair, the makeup, the jewelry, so that the sweater is seen as a deliberate choice and not a lazy one. Stylish women are never lazy.

15.

Caftan

T HE CAFTAN IS ALL ABOUT lounging and luxury. Banish the images of Mrs. Roper in *Three's Company* or your grandmother in Miami. These are not your grandmother's caftans we're talking about. We are talking Talitha Getty in Marrakech. Cristiana Brandolini in Venice. Diana Vreeland at her ruby-red apartment in Manhattan. It's so low-key and so unapologetically antifashion that it has once again become one of the most fashionable items in the world.

You'll find the best designer caftans—Muriel Brandolini (Cristiana's daughter-in-law), Allegra Hicks, Yves Saint Laurent Rive Gauche—at the high-end stores. If you want the real deal, go to an ethnic shop, where you can find the traditional Moroccan or Indian versions. Either way, paired with a string of beads and some flat shoes, the caftan remains the epitome of jet-set chic. Wear it over your bathing suit and with a pair of flip-flops. Or dress it up with a high metallic sandal and a pile of exotic bangles. Play around with it. Look at the old fashion photographs from the '60s and '70s, and take notice of style icons like Babe Paley and Marella Agnelli. These women wore the caftan the way it is meant to be worn.

SUNSHINE
GLAMOUR

The caftan (or *kaftan*) dates back to the four-teenth century and has always been a staple in Mid- to Far Eastern countries, where the climates demand light, cool clothing. In the 1960s and '70s, when the West became obsessed with all things Eastern, the caftan made its way to mainstream fashion. Yves Saint Laurent became enamored with Marrakech and was the first to reinvent the traditional caftan, make it high fashion, and send it down the runway. With that, centuries-old dress became the epitome of 1970s boho chic. Both the jet set and the college crowd adopted the caftan; it became the favored uniform to wear while sitting on a bean bag, sparking up, and discussing Eastern philosophy.

WHAT'S IN A NAME ...

- **Caftan:** Turkish origin. A long cloak, with or without sleeves. Usually long and voluminous; most often made from linen or silk.
- **Djellaba:** Egyptian/Arab origin. A long, flowing robe, traditionally worn by men in the Middle East.
- **Tunic:** Greco-Roman origin. A simple, slip-on garment. Usually knee-length, but can be shorter (especially the modern tunic top; Google *Tory Burch*).

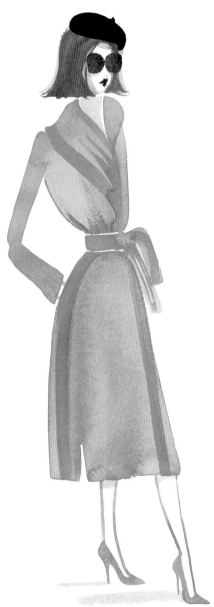

16.
Camel Coat

TRUE CLASSIC COAT that looks both elegant and expensive if the color is right (a golden tan with red to light brown undertones). The camel coat has become the ultimate uptown coat that women will wear to give their jeans an upscale air. It also brings an urbane sensibility to an all-white or all-black outfit. But this coat is not just for the sophisticated set. Every girl should have a camel coat for those winter days when she needs alternatives to the black coat. And for those nights when she feels like playing the uptown girl.

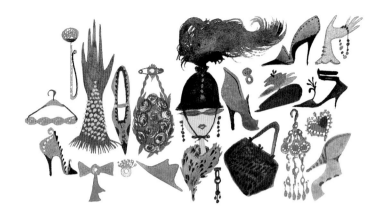

AH, THE LUXURY . . .

- Camel is a warm, rich color that is great to use in combination with black, white, brown.
- Calvin Klein, Ralph Lauren, and Michael Kors always make great versions.
- If you want to invest, go for genius camel hair.

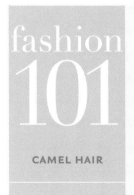

fashion 101

CAMEL HAIR

Camel hair is a precious fabric that is made from the underhair of a camel. The gatherers follow the camel herds collecting hairs, which spontaneously fall. The most prized hairs come from Mongolia and the Persian Gulf. Camel hair is often blended with wool to cut cost. A blend of camel hair and another fiber will be indicated on the label; if the item is made of pure camel hair, there will likely be a picture of a camel on the label. Always read the fine print.

17.

Cape

‹∞›

I T IS A GARMENT often associated with eccentrics and su-per-heroes, but the cape can be very elegant and practical. The cape is bold, mysterious, and powerful. There is a reason Superman and Dracula are such big fans. It is the perfect way to add drama, hides a multitude of flaws, and is a great option to pair with an evening dress. It can be knit, wool, velvet, cashmere, or fur. As global warming progresses and makes the weather as unpredictable as can be, the capes will come out of the closet a lot more. Thankfully. Living in a world without capes would be a dull world indeed.

CAPE FEAR

- Keep everything else tight to the body. A cape looks best when the layer underneath is tailored. Baggy layers underneath the cape take away the cosmopolitan cachet you are going for.
- For a more formal evening option, use a capelet to top off your dress.

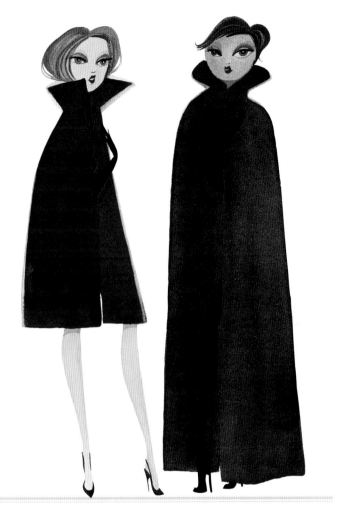

Go in peace, my daughter.
And remember that, in a world of ordinary mortals,
you are a Wonder Woman.

QUEEN HIPPOLYTE

18.

Cashmere Sweater

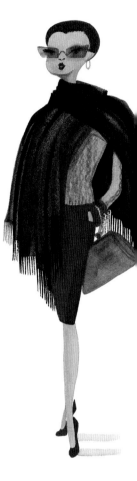

WOMEN FIRST BEGAN craving cashmere in 1937, when Lana Turner wore her tight cashmere sweater in the film *They Won't Forget*. And nobody did forget that sweater. From that moment, women began their cashmere collections.

It is advisable to have as many as possible in as many versions as possible: a cardigan, a turtleneck, a crewneck, a V-neck, a wrap, etc. The massive appeal of cashmere is the silken, featherlight feel that will always make you feel luxe. It is also, ounce for ounce, the warmest of natural fibers, so it provides coziness without bulk.

Luxury must be comfortable,
otherwise it is not luxury.

COCO CHANEL

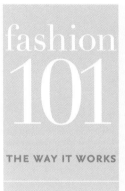

fashion
101

THE WAY IT WORKS

Cashmere wool is spun from the fibers of the cashmere goat. The goats are raised mostly in Mongolia and China. Once the fibers are collected, they are sent mostly to Italy or Scotland to be spun into yarn and knitted into sweaters

SHOPPING FOR CASHMERE

- Let yourself spend a little. You can find cashmere at any price point, but if you want quality that will last, be prepared to spend at least $200.
- For summer-weight cashmere, look for a cashmere blend with silk.
- The higher the ply, the warmer the sweater (it will also be more expensive). If you live in Vermont go for a higher ply, and if you live in Florida go for a lower one.

19.
Charm Bracelet

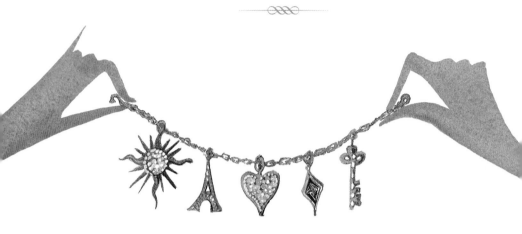

WHEN A CHARM BRACELET is added onto charm by charm, it can be the most precious piece of jewelry in your collection. Designers have begun to issue ready-made versions, but the best charm bracelets are pure expressions of your creativity. They are something you add to as the years go by, and each charm has a meaning, a milestone, or a memory to go along with it. It is like a diary, but worn on your wrist or tucked in your jewelry box and waiting for the day you can pass it down. The greatest part of the charm bracelet is that when you are older, it will remind you of moments in your life, and you will be able to tell your children and grandchildren what each charm means.

CHARMED

- A charm bracelet is a very personal piece that you can start at any time in your life. It is a wonderful thing to start when you hit a milestone— graduating high school, entering college, getting married, having a child—so that it will remind you of those specific years.
- Consider having several charm bracelets and giving each one a theme, or have one charm bracelet and gradually build upon it.
- It makes a beautiful gift, and you can pass down an entirely built charm bracelet, or a starter with a few charms that you have picked out. Then the recipient can build from there.
- This is a great item to shop for vintage and looks much more authentic when some of the pieces are new and some are older. Don't get too stuffy about it.

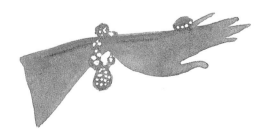

fashion 101

CHARMING

Charm bracelets date back to the ancient Egyptians. They used them to ward off evil spirits and show their status. But the main function of the charm bracelet for the Egyptian was to be a sort of ID tag to help the gods place each person in their proper status level on the other side and to reunite them with all of their belongings. Think of it as a boarding pass for the afterlife.

CHARM BRACELETS I'D LIKE TO SEE

- **Marlene Dietrich:** She had one made out of poker chips, given to her by Frank Sinatra. And one that had religious figures and good-luck symbols—she was convinced it kept her safe when flying.
- **Elizabeth Taylor:** She had many—one had all heart charms signifying her love of children, friends . . . and husbands.
- **Mrs. Walt Disney:** Had a charm bracelet from Walt with twenty-two miniature Oscars, signifying how many Oscars he had won.

- Doyle & Doyle: A jewelry store on the Lower East Side of Manhattan that carries handpicked antique and estate jewels at reasonable prices.
- C.H.A.R.M: A company with a huge collection of vintage-inspired charms. There are sure to be pieces that represent every facet of your life, no matter what your personality.
- Louis Vuitton charm bracelets: LV has brought high fashion to the charm bracelet. The house makes charms based on the theme of travel, which cost a pretty penny but are oh-so-gorgeous.

I really think that American gentlemen are the best after all, because kissing your hand may make you feel very good, but a diamond-and-sapphire bracelet lasts forever.

ANITA LOOS

20

Clutch

⎯⎯∞∞⎯⎯

THE CLUTCH IS the best companion for an evening out. It will not get in the way of your look and only support your stylish efforts. Take advantage. The clutch is the one item that will let you show off your sense of whimsy, your sense of glamour. They come in all shapes, sizes, colors, and materials. A clutch adds excitement to a black outfit. Try out beaded, python skin, bright colors, brocade, silk/satin versions. It's all fair game here. Have fun! On a practical level (if we must), make sure that the bag will fit all of your essentials— lipstick, cash, cell phone, credit card. And then make sure that it will fit snugly under your arm, because perhaps the best aspect of the clutch is that it will leave your hands free to meet, greet, hold drinks, tell stories, and show off your Cocktail Ring (see #21).

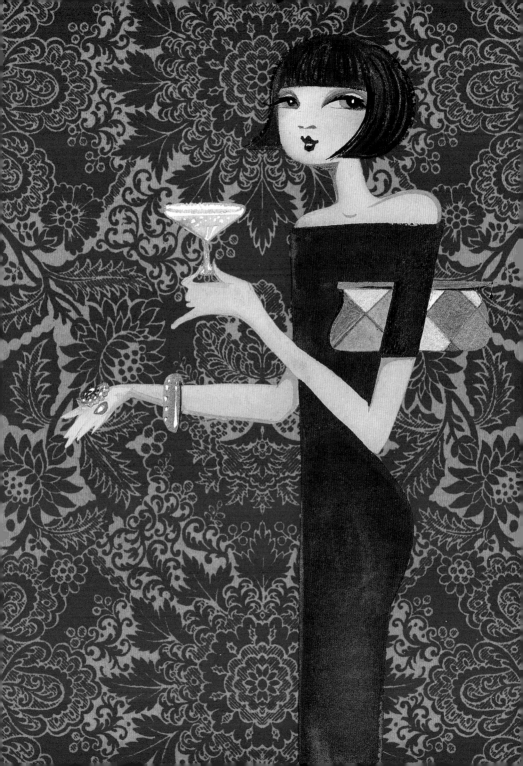

THE CLUTCH PLAY

- Try out something that you normally shy away from: jewels, metallics, wood, shagreen (sharkskin, galuchat), or horn.
- This is a perfect item to pick up on your travels. In Asia and Thailand, they make really beautiful wood boxes. In the Philippines you can find them in woven silver cloth. Anywhere you go, you are sure to find a unique version.
- Always have one in gold and one in silver for evening.
- If you don't want to spend a fortune, look for them in ethnic shops, flea markets, and vintage stores. Or ask Grandma if she has one you can steal.
- Look at it as a piece of jewelry. It should add to the outfit and make a statement.

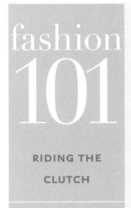

fashion 101

RIDING THE CLUTCH

The idea of the clutch purse originated in the Victorian era, when proper ladies carried small, decorative bags in order to store their handkerchiefs and smelling salts. It wasn't until World War II that the clutch became a mainstream fashion staple. Because of the rationing during the war, everything had to be downsized and the clutch became the bag of choice. When the rationing ended, women refused to let go of the clutch, and it is now an essential item in every chic woman's wardrobe.

THE INSIDE TRACK:
FASHION EDITOR FAVORITES

- Elsa Peretti clutch for Tiffany: If you ever come across one of these clutches in silver, beg, borrow, or steal it. I am still trying to get my hands on one.
- Judith Leiber animal clutches: I am not proposing you carry an animal around on a regular basis, but it is great for those occasions when you want to add a little whimsy to your look.
- Nancy Gonzalez: Makes a box clutch in every color of the crocodile rainbow (see Exotic Skin Bag, #31, for more info).
- Calvin Klein Box clutch: It is plain and minimalist—pure Calvin—and will be here season after season.
- Bottega Veneta Knot: Woven bag with a knot clasp. It costs a fortune, but a girl can dream.
- VBH Envelope clutch: My favorite. It is a simple and elegant bag available in leather or exotic skin.
- R & Y Augousti: Specializes in unique shagreen designs.

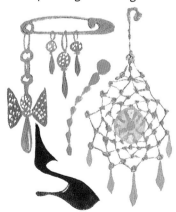

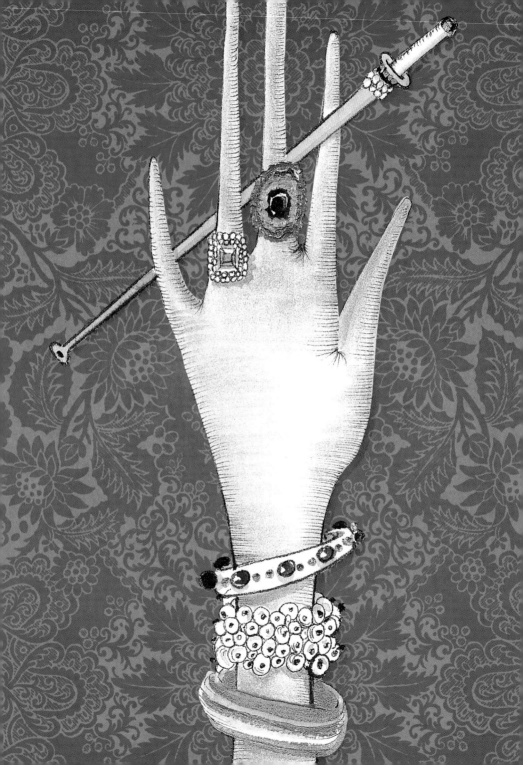

21.
Cocktail Ring

AVING IT AROUND at the party when you are telling a story, flashing it as you pose on the red carpet, twirling it around when you feel like playing shy—hands down, a cocktail ring is one of the best ways to show that you've got style. It's all about size and making a statement. And a great cocktail ring does not have to be real—in some cases, a big vintage fake is even preferred. The wealthiest women will admit that wearing a piece of costume jewelry is almost better than wearing a big, expensive heirloom. The cachet of a cocktail ring is not about the cost. It's about being bold, daring, and adventurous.

FUN FACT

The term "cocktail ring" emerged during Prohibition, when women would wear large, bold rings to illegal cocktail parties. A woman would flit her hand around, drawing attention to the bauble, to let you know that not only was she drinking illegally, she was doing it with style.

FASHION EDITOR FAVORITES

CLASSIC

- Victoire de Castellane for Christian Dior: A witty and genius designer with a wild imagination. Her creations are bold, glamorous, witty, and flamboyant. She says, "I like things to be over-the-top. . . . Average doesn't interest me at all." A good rule of thumb to keep in mind in regard to the cocktail ring!
- H. Stern: Makes big rings of semiprecious stones. A favorite of top celebrities, but H. Stern always introduces some rings at a lower price point for the younger client.
- Tony Duquette: Extravagant gemstone rings. Duquette was a lavish interior designer who brought flash and flamboyance to his jewelry designs.
- Stephen Dweck: Loved for his rings and jewelry inspired by art and nature. He collects stones from all over the world to create one-of-a-kind pieces.
- David Webb: Trademarks of a David Webb are exciting colors, bold designs, and often exotic animals (think big, gold, cougar-shaped ring with emerald eyes). These are all heirloom-quality jewels.

MODERN TAKES

- Loree Rodkin: Huge punk/medieval-style rings that go over the knuckle. For the rocker chick (the *very rich* rocker chick).
- Chrome Hearts: Silver rings with gothic motifs.
- Stephen Webster: The ring for the bad girls. Designs include skulls, skeletons, and ironic inscriptions.

KENNETH JAY LANE, THE BIG FAKE

Kenneth Jay Lane is the costume jewelry king. For every ring mentioned above, he has a great knockoff version. Women have always loved him. Everyone from Jackie O to Audrey Hepburn to Diana Vreeland were big fans. He has been successful for decades, and his faux jewels are now coveted as if they were real. Must-haves, for sure.

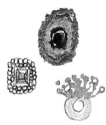

RING A DING DING!

WHEN LOOKING FOR A COCKTAIL RING:

- SIZE MATTERS: Go big or go home. Go for five carats or more. The bigger and bolder, the better.
- FAKING IT IS FINE: Even the wealthiest women do it.
- BE DRAMATIC: The cocktail ring is meant to make a statement, start a conversation, and represent a piece of your personality.

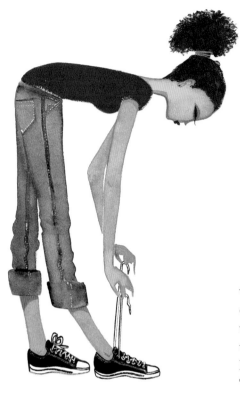

22

Converse

T HE ULTIMATE cool-kid sneaker. This is the shoe that the models are always wearing when they walk out of shoots and that every downtown girl wears in her down-time. It makes them look as though they aren't trying too hard and have not overthought their look. They wear them with skirts or skinny jeans and plain white T-shirts. Each time I see them, I am always enamored by their kick-back style.

Converse has become famous for its collaborations with artists. For its 100th birthday, the company launched the Red Converse 1HUND(RED) initiative to help eliminate AIDS in Africa. The 1HUND(RED) is a yearlong global project in which Converse commissioned one hundred musicians and graphic and graffiti artists from all over the world to create one-of-a-kind sneaker designs. The initiative includes a "Make Mine Red" platform that lets the customer use custom colors and patterns to create a personalized pair. Just another indication of how in touch Converse is with the hip, downtown crowd.

fashion
101

CONVERSE

Converse were created as a basketball shoe almost a hundred years ago and remained an athletic shoe until the '50s, when the Beach Boys, James Dean, and Elvis started sporting them on stage and film. American teenagers began wearing them too, and Converse became more than just a basketball shoe. In the 1960s, the company capitalized on their youth following and began producing Converse in different colors (they used to be available only in black and white) and created the Oxford low-cut version, which remains a fan favorite. Today, they are found next to Louboutins and Manolos in women's closets.

FUN FACTS

- **60% OF AMERICANS** claim to have owned at least one pair of Converse in their lives.
- **CONVERSE HIGH-TOPS** are also called Chuck Taylors, because in 1918, a high-school basketball star, Chuck Taylor, began wearing them. He later promoted and lent his name to the sneakers.

23.
Cosmetics Bag

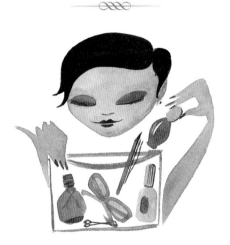

I T MAY SEEM LIKE an insignificant accessory, but any woman on the go will tell you that this is the one item she would be lost without. Some women go really high-end (Prada, Vuitton, Bottega Veneta, Tod's); others keep it simple (LeSportsac or MAC). If you buy a good-looking one in satin or velvet, it can double up as a clutch, especially when traveling. I have the satin Prada version in four colors, and when I am in a pinch, I use them for clutches, receipt holders, etc.

But—let's be honest—in this case, it's what's on the inside that really counts (although you do want it to look nice when you pull it out of your bag).

On sets and shoots, I am always vaguely curious about what's inside everyone's cosmetics bag. Here is a peek inside mine.

- LA ROCHE POSAY SUNSCREEN: An insider secret for years, this sunscreen contains a special ingredient, mexoryl, that protects against UVA and UVB rays.
- KIEHL'S LIP BALM: Inexpensive, fragrance-free, addictive.
- GUERLAIN BRONZING POWDER: Luminous powder with iridescent highlights that enhance the face and make you look sun-kissed.
- NIVEA SUN OIL SPRAY: Instantly makes legs look thinner and more toned.
- KÉRASTASE HAIR DROPS: Makes hair smooth, shiny, and stronger.
- MARIO BADESCU DRYING LOTION: Zaps blemishes overnight.
- HELENA RUBINSTEIN FORCE C CREAM: Every model and makeup artist uses this cream.
- MAYBELLINE GREAT LASH MASCARA: The pink tube with the green top.
- MAC EYE SHADOW: Great colors, blends perfectly, and lasts all day.
- BOBBI BROWN LONG-WEAR EYELINER: This gel eyeliner goes on easy, can be natural or dramatic, and actually lasts.
- TWEEZERMAN TWEEZERS: Gets the hair every time!
- SHU UEMURA EYELASH CURLER: The iconic and standard curler delivers the perfect curl to make your eyes pop.

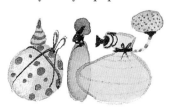

There are no ugly women, only lazy ones.

HELENA RUBINSTEIN

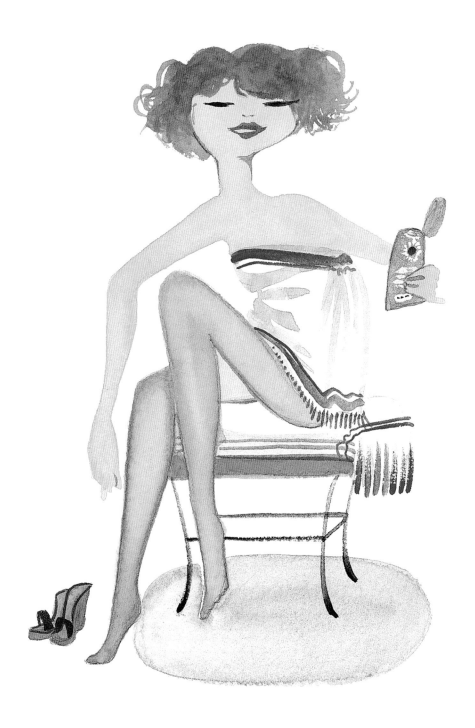

24.

Cowboy Boots

I F YOU'RE FROM A PLACE where cowboy boots are part of the landscape, then you know how to wear them. But those of us who were not born down South or out West have to tread lightly at first. The rule of thumb is there is no rule of thumb. They are just as acceptable with cocktail dresses as they are with jeans and a T-shirt. But the cocktail dress and cowboy boot is hard to pull off if you weren't born with a pair of Tony Lamas on your feet. If it's your first foray into the cowboy boot arena, I'd start with a Hanes T-shirt and your favorite pair of Levi's (jeans *over* the boots always!). Then, when you've got the swagger down, pair them with a flowy white sundress and some funky jewelry or a peasant skirt and a jean jacket. The cocktail dress takes a bit of experience; perhaps it can best be pulled off down South or out West. And personally, I'm leaving the *Dukes of Hazzard* look to Miss Daisy, but that's just me.

FUN FACT

Cowboy boots were "invented" when an in-genious cowboy brought his cavalry boots to a shoemaker and asked him to make the toe pointed so that he could get his foot in and out of the stirrups easier.

SADDLE UP

- If you want to get that real cowgirl swagger, go for the real Texas deal—either Tony Lama or Lucchese (pronounced *loo-CAY-see*). Texans swear by these two designers, and in a state where there are bootmakers on every corner and several pairs of boots are in every woman's closet, I'm going to take Texans at their word. Both Tony Lama and Lucchese are based out of El Paso.
- Spend a little money. A good pair of boots will become a part of you. After you've worn them long enough, they'll be some of the most comfortable shoes in your closet.
- Most important, you have to beat them up. Any cowgirl will tell you: You just can't get that swagger in a brand-new boot.

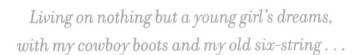

Living on nothing but a young girl's dreams,
with my cowboy boots and my old six-string . . .

MARY CHAPIN CARPENTER

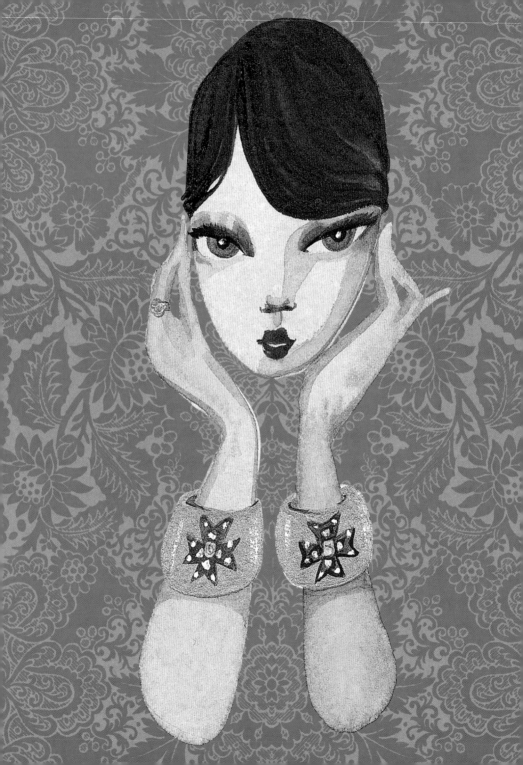

25

Cuff

THE CUFF IS the one bracelet that is always, always on the runway. Because of its heft, it always makes a statement and never goes unnoticed. Which is why it is also a piece that is often used to assert or proclaim someone's personal style. The uptown girl wears a platinum or diamond version. The bohemian girl wears leather or wood. The rocker chick goes for black leather with studs. It is a bold item that can add edge to an otherwise demure outfit or a touch of glamour to an otherwise casual look.

The four classic materials are ebony, silver, Lucite, and wood. Though they are also found in diamond, leather, platinum, etc.

YOU'VE GOT THE RIGHT CUFF, BABY

- Try mixing precious and semiprecious cuffs on one arm.
- Consider mixing them in with your bangles.
- To channel your inner Wonder Woman, throw a cuff on each arm.

FASHION EDITOR FAVORITES

- Hermès Collier de Chien: A leather cuff that is both punk and posh. A cult item.
- Kara Ross: An array of unique and special pieces that refuse to be ignored.
- Robert Lee Morris: Morris often collaborates with designers to make iconic, covetable pieces.
- David Webb: The designer who started the animal bracelet (see Cocktail Ring, #21).
- John Hardy: Balinese-inspired cuffs. The designer still uses ancient Balinese design techniques.
- Patricia von Musulin: Modern, sculptural designs that will be modern 100 years from now.
- Elsa Peretti: The classic Wave cuff from Tiffany.
- Chanel: From the house that first popularized costume jewelry—these cuffs are iconic.

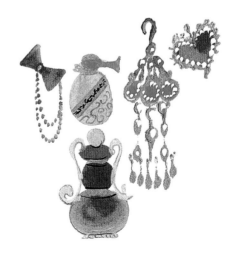

CLOSET OBSESSION: **VERDURA CUFF**

Those iconic cuffs with the bejeweled Maltese cross are from Verdura. Oh-so-exquisite (and oh-so-expensive). Though Coco Chanel is sometimes credited with creating the Verdura cuff, they were actually the brainchild of Fulco di Verdura. But Mme did have her influence. She had a lot of lovers who gave her a lot of jewelry, which she asked Verdura to reset. He came up with the cuff, and Chanel was enchanted by his bizarre and surreal style. She wore the cuffs everywhere, making them one of her trademarks. Today Verdura cuffs are available in jade, carnelian, green jade, sandalwood, ebony, and walnut. Since they begin at $12,500, it's probably best to seek out a costume version.

I can resist everything except temptation.

OSCAR WILDE

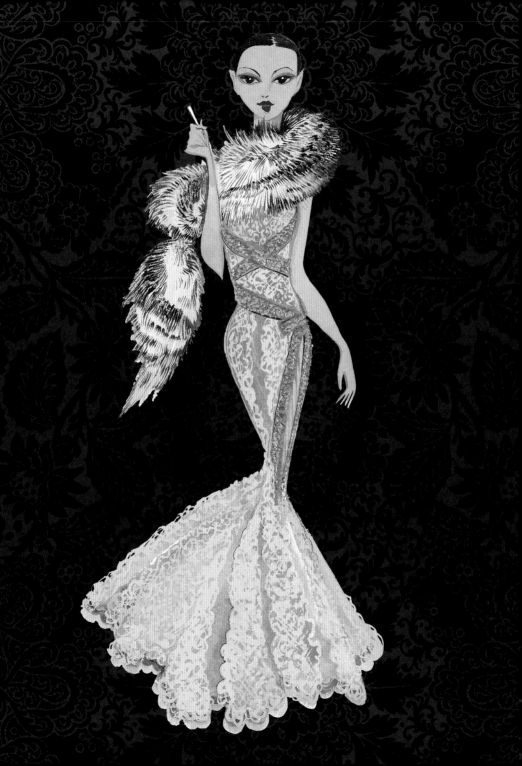

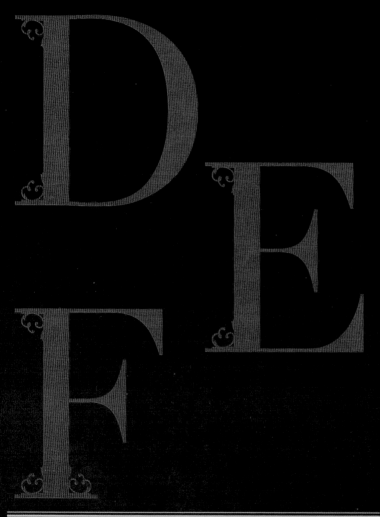

26.

Denim Jacket

⸺◦∞◦⸺

THE EBBS AND FLOWS of the denim jacket clearly reveal how fashion reinvents itself decade after decade. Just when you think it is a relic, the good old denim jacket makes its comeback. In the '50s, it was popularized by the greasers. And in the '60s and '70s, Janis Joplin and the hippies laid their claim, wearing it to peace protests and rock festivals (sometimes even successfully pulling it off with a pair of jeans), and the greasers were all but forgotten. Then, in the '80s, everyone wanted in on the jacket—the hair bands, the punks, the princesses (armed with their bedazzlers), and everyone in between. It became so synonymous with the decade that at '80s parties across America there was sure to be a solid denim-jacket contingent. And in the '90s, Ralph Lauren borrowed the jacket out of the hands of the crazy kids, paired it with long prairie skirts, cowboy boots, and turquoise jewelry, and it suddenly seemed as though it was always meant to be worn that way. Now, when we see them cropped and shrunken on the models and actresses of the moment, we abandon all notions of the past decades and set out to stake our claim on the old classic once again.

BEEN THERE,
DENIM THAT

- Be extreme. It should either be really dark or really worn out.
- Buy it a size too small or find a really fitted model.
- In general, don't wear it with another piece of blue denim. The jean tuxedo is strictly for the cowboys. Who actually rodeo and herd cattle. But a blue jean jacket with white jeans is a definite yes!
- Every jean maker should have a version, but a few great sources include Levis, A.P.C., Diesel, Marc by Marc Jacobs. And of course, the vintage shops.

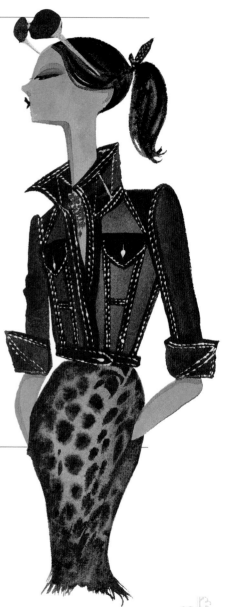

27.

Diamond Studs

BEST WHEN LARGE, real, and received as a gift. But large, fake, and self-purchased do the job, too (if you lose one, you won't want to kill yourself). They are a perfect everyday earring, as they add a bit of sparkle without being obnoxiously in-your-face about it. There are not many outfits that the diamond stud doesn't get along with.

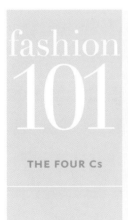

fashion 101

THE FOUR Cs

- **Color:** The most valued white diamonds are colorless or nearly colorless.
- **Cut:** Refers to how skillfully the diamond has been faceted, not the shape. It should be symmetrical and proportional.
- **Clarity:** The most valuable diamonds are, of course, flawless. Imperfections on the surface are called blemishes, and internal fractures are called inclusions.
- **Carat:** The measure of the diamond's weight. One carat equals 200 milligrams.

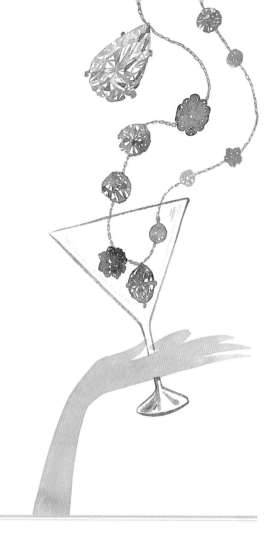

No gold digging for me . . . I take diamonds.

MAE WEST

28.
Driving Shoe

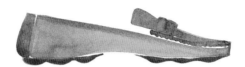

A DRIVING SHOE means one thing: leisure. It is almost always seen on long plane rides and in weekends on Nantucket. It is supremely comfortable and is the more fashionable option to the loafer. They always look amazing when worn with white jeans or khakis and a crisp Man's White Shirt (see #53)—which makes such a fantastically WASP-chic outfit. It was a man's shoe first, and they generally wore them to drive to black ties, changing their shoes when they arrived. If you want to be literal about things, I guess you could do that—in general, I suggest taxis. Who can fit a pair of driving shoes into her clutch?

Also called the car shoe, it is a light shoe with its roots in the loafer. The car shoe is differentiated by the tiny rubber gussets on the soles, which were intended for traction when driving. The first car shoe was patented in 1963 by Gianni Mostile, who had a passion for both shoes and race cars. Style icons such as JFK and Roberto Rossellini began car shoes as streetwear.

SOLE SISTERS

- Try them in bright, bold colors in the summer.
- Keep the logos or hardware to a minimum.
- Look for unusual animal prints or exotic skins.
- To be indulgent, get them in butterscotch suede. They look amazing with tan legs.
- Remember: They look better aged.

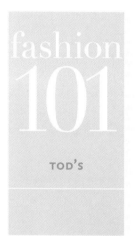

fashion 101

TOD'S

Tod's, the Italian company known for their iconic luxury driving shoe, actually owes a debt of gratitude to good old American preppy elegance. The son of a renowned cobbler, Diego Della Valle first visited America in 1978, and was taken with how Americans "weekended" in chic but casual clothes. "On the weekends, the U.S. was casual," he said. "In Italy, the weekend was very formal. I came to understand that weekends are about free time, and that one could wear high quality, tasteful products that weren't so formal." He then came up with the idea for a casual luxury shoe, and the classic Tod's driving shoe was born.

FUN FACT

The name J.P. Tod's was taken out of the 1978 Boston telephone directory because it sounded good in all languages.

29.

Espadrilles

HE ULTIMATE summer shoe. When the impossible happens and the winter turns to summer in a matter of twenty-four hours, one must have a pair of espadrilles to wear with a sundress, your favorite white jeans, or a caftan. The espadrille, a shoe of Spanish and Portuguese origin, is characterized by a sole made from twisted cord sewn on sturdy cloth. The flat espadrille had originally been a shoe of peasants, warriors, and Mediterranean fishermen. Today's espadrilles are high-heeled and would not fare well in warfare or on serious fishing trips. Christian Louboutin makes the ultimate fashion version, which remain in highly coveted style season after season.

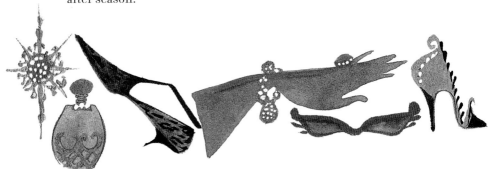

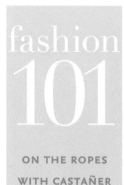

fashion
101

ON THE ROPES

WITH CASTAÑER

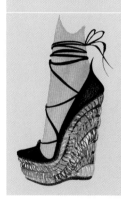

Espadrilles did not go high fashion or high-heeled until the 1960s, when Yves Saint Laurent met up with Isabel Castañer at a trade fair in Paris. The now-famous Spanish Castañer shoe company had been making espadrilles since 1776, but it was on the point of closing its doors. There was no longer a market for the espadrille, which started out as a humble flat shoe for peasants and country folk. Along came Yves Saint Laurent, who asked Castañer if they could make an espadrille with a high heel. That request saved the company. Nobody had ever thought of a high-heeled espadrille before, but as soon as it hit the market, the shoe took off. Today, the label is legendary in Spain and around the world. It is also clearly the favorite among the fashion set, as Yves Saint Laurent, Louis Vuitton, and Donna Karan all commission Castañer to manufacture their espadrilles.

I just want to let them know they didn't break me.

MOLLY RINGWALD IN *PRETTY IN PINK*

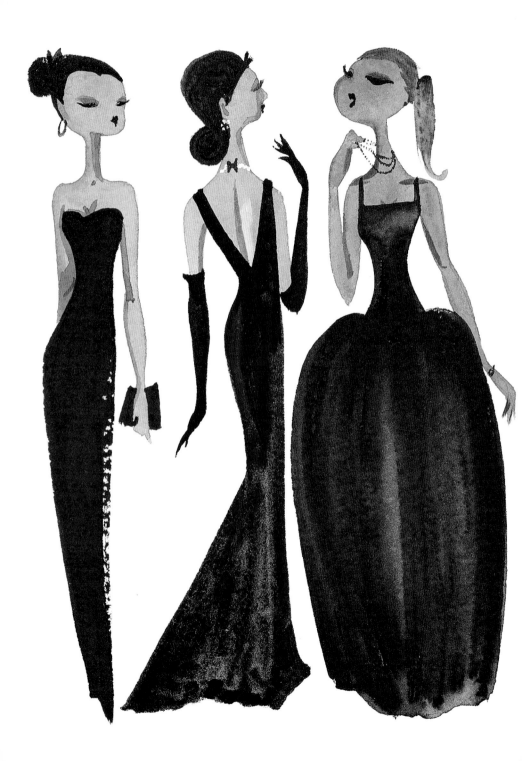

30.
Evening Gown

Watching famous women on the red carpet wear their evening gowns has become a sort of sport. We all sit there and comment, judge, and praise or deify. But when the situation is turned on us, when we are the ones who have to go somewhere that requires an evening gown, we often enter into a state of terror. This is why you should buy an evening gown when you do not need it. Typically, we search for an evening gown only when we have somewhere to go. Then we are in the torturous situation of the *under-pressure-evening-gown-hunt*. A few hours into the search, we will usually throw our hands up in defeat and spend too much on a dress we are not even that crazy about.

The smarter girl never passes a sale rack without looking at the evening gowns. If she sees one she loves, she buys it. It does not matter that she has no black-tie events in her future. She knows that the invite will come—and when it does, it's best to have an evening gown waiting in the wings.

THE CLASSIC OPTIONS FOR EACH BODY TYPE
- STRAPLESS: If your chest and arms are your best feature.
- COLUMN: For the tall and thin.
- BIAS-CUT: For the curvy, feminine body.
- GODDESS: For everyone.

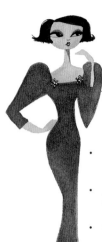

THE GREAT GOWN SEARCH

- Opt for a year-round fabric: chiffon, lightweight crepe, or lightweight silk or satin.
- Avoid any details that will make the dress go out of style. Too much beading, ruffles, too many colors, prints.
- Choose a dark or neutral color that can be worn over and over again (just change your accessories each time).
- The most figure-flattering option: a bias-cut gown in chiffon or satin (bias is a cut that follows the line of the body and is easier to wear than a straight-cut dress).

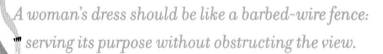

A woman's dress should be like a barbed-wire fence: serving its purpose without obstructing the view.

SOPHIA LOREN

31

Exotic Skin Bag

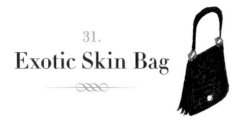

E VERYTHING ELSE can be kept classic—the exotic skin bag is happy to carry the whole look. The appeal of an exotic skin bag is that it will make you look instantly luxe. Grab your crocodile tote or a snakeskin clutch, and *voilà*—you are the envy of women everywhere. And, best of all, not one of those women will ever have the same exact bag that you are carrying. It is assuredly unique, because the patterns, lines, and textures of the skin will never be the same. An exotic skin bag is the anti-"It" bag, which is reason enough to buy two.

THE WEAR, THE WHAT, AND THE WHY

- A great item to search for at vintage shows or in vintage shops. You can get them at a third of the price!
- The three skins that will never go out of style: crocodile, snakeskin, and ostrich.
- If you need justification for spending the money on an exotic skin (they don't come cheap!), just remember that you will have this bag forever.

CLOSET OBSESSION: **NANCY GONZALEZ**

Nancy Gonzalez makes some of my favorite exotic skin bags. Though the designs are classic, there are clear elements of fun (bold colors, woven crocodile and cobra, etc.). Best of all, in a label-obsessed world, there is no logo. The skin speaks for itself. It is high quality and the designs are never trendy, so you can pull it out season after season and it never gets tired. Because it is both classic and fun, you'll find these skins in the hands of both sophisticated older women and hip young fashion girls.

Some people think luxury is the opposite of poverty.
It is not. It is the opposite of vulgarity.

COCO CHANEL

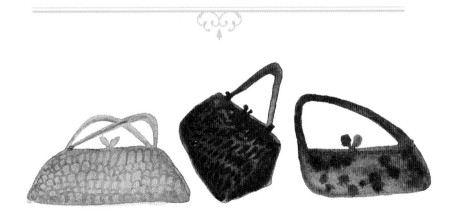

32.

Fishnets

FISHNETS WERE ORIGINALLY worn only by questionable women in dark, dank bars, but in the '20s, they were brought out into the light by the intrepid flappers. Marlene Dietrich made these all the rage. They are most powerful when just a little flicker of the fishnet is shown (a few inches at the knee, a centimeter at the peep toe). Teasing with fishnets is incredibly sexy and intriguing. It makes one wonder what else is underneath. A little bit of Marlene Dietrich? A touch of Dita Von Teese? But if the entire leg of fishnets is showing with too short a skirt and too high a heel, all the intrigue is gone. We all know what kind of woman that is. And you don't want to be her.

Basically, I'm the girl your mother warned you about.

DITA VON TEESE

GOING FISHIN'

Fishnets are supersexy when done right, supertawdry when done wrong. To stay on the right side of the line, make sure you:

- CHOOSE A FINE MESH. Keep it between an eighth and a quarter of an inch. The smaller, the better.
- PAIR WITH SOPHISTICATED CLOTHING. Try a blouse with a pencil skirt or pants and a flicker of fishnet at the feet.
- TRY IT IN A NUDE.
- DON'T LET TOO MUCH SHOW. A peek of fishnet at the ankle, when you are wearing tailored trousers, can go much further than showing an entire leg of fishnet with high heels and a short skirt.

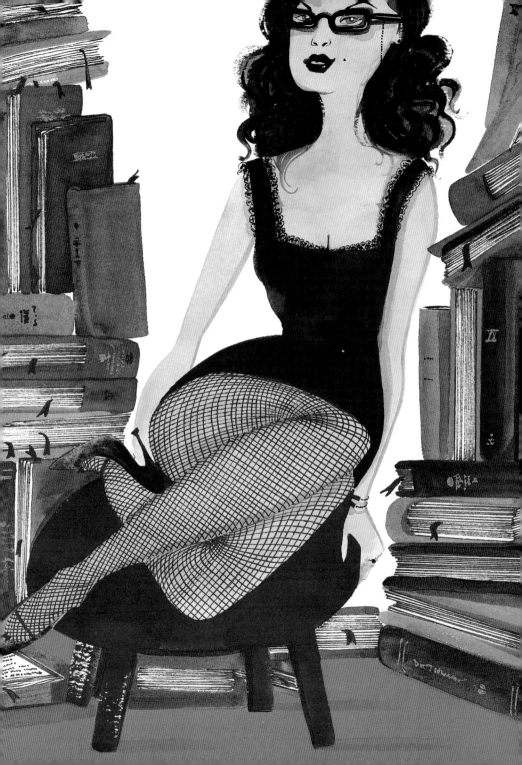

33

Frye Harness Boot

I N THE '60S, women began to wear Frye boots in clear and bold defiance of restrictive 1950s femininity. They were a boot that meant strength and power, which women were intent on claiming at the time. High heels took a backseat to these clunky, chunky boots. Every woman seemed to have a pair, and they were such an iconic part of the decade that when the Smithsonian Institution was searching for items to represent 1960s America, they chose a pair of Fryes. And perhaps it is because women have not let go of our strength and power, we have also never let go of this big, clunky boot. At first glance, it seems to have nothing to do with fashion. But the Frye boot asserts an element of our personality that says we are unwilling to always be so fragile and feminine—sometimes we want to be flat-out kickass. And that has everything to do with fashion.

FRYE GIRL

- The older and more beat up they are, the better.
- Wear them with jeans tucked in or with dresses and a Boyfriend Cardigan (see #12).

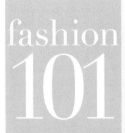

fashion
101

FRYE BOOTS

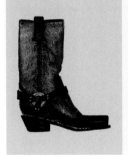

The Frye Company has a long and illustrious history. It was founded in 1863 and is the oldest continuously operated shoe company in the United States. Frye boots were worn by soldiers for both sides of the Civil War, pioneers going West in the late 1800s, Teddy Roosevelt, General Patton, and servicemen in World Wars I and II. They were a completely functional shoe, but it was in the '60s that the Frye boot became a fashion item.

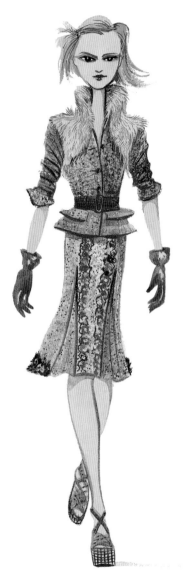

34.

Fur

⌬

WHETHER YOU DECIDE TO GO real or fake is entirely up to you. Just make sure it's fabulous either way. It has to be glamorous and gorgeous—otherwise, it's pointless!

IF YOU GO REAL

The five that I prefer, in order of price and luxe factor, are: sable, chinchilla, mink, Astrakhan/broadtail, and Orylag. In Italy, where the well-to-do girls all receive their first fur on their eighteenth birthday, the women can tell you the much more blown-out hierarchy. The Italians collect their furs like the French collect their scarves and Americans collect their jeans, so they can unapologetically tell you how to best wear fur. With everything. It adds the glam factor to jeans, evening gowns, dresses, etc. There is nothing that fur does not play well with.

GREAT FINDS AT: J. Mendel, Fendi, Dennis Basso, vintage shops

fashion
101

FUR EVER

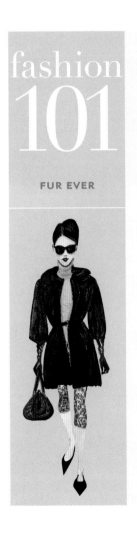

- **Sable:** If you have endless funds, this is your fur. It is extraordinarily beautiful with an incredible silvery sheen due to its lack of pigmentation in the tips of the fur. Before oil was discovered, sable was considered "black gold," and it remains as precious today as it was in ancient times.

- **Chinchilla:** A soft, velvety fur that is both light and voluptuous. It sways and changes colors with each gust of the wind and movement of the body. The changing colors range from silver-white, gray-blue, pearl gray, rose-beige, and black. It is a mark and marvel of luxury and high fashion.

- **Mink:** Perhaps the most popular fur. It is both soft and glossy, and the colors range all the way from white to dark brown and black. It is a fur that offers fashion designers a large number of creative options, and is thus found in all sorts of mutations.

- **Astrakhan/Broadtail:** Both are made from Persian lamb and are the fur of choice for the bohemian girls. Astrakhan has a coarse, loose curl that provides for a unique design. Broadtail has a beautiful, silky, moiré effect because the curl has not yet developed.

- **Orylag:** Orylag is a rabbit fur that is dyed to look like it is the more expensive chinchilla. It feels and looks like chinchilla, and only a real connoisseur can tell the difference.

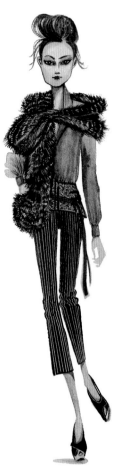

CLOSET OBSESSION:
FUR STOLES

Ladies, we have to talk. I understand it is hard to match a stylish coat to an evening dress. But a day coat looks horrid with eveningwear and no coat at all looks silly when it is freezing out! This is where a beautiful fur stole comes into play. Every girl should have one. It fills a multitude of wardrobe holes. It always adds Hollywood glamour to an evening dress. And it will make you look *finished* . . . like you haven't forgotten your coat in the cab.

IF YOU GO FAUX

The huge mistake when going faux is to try to buy furs that look like the real thing. No! No! Google *Prada's Fake Classic Fall 2007*. Look at how Prada does not try to make their furs imitate the real thing, instead giving them a life and a beauty all their own, dyeing them in shocking oranges or creating big, white, impossibly puffy coats. It is so clear that they are fake, which makes them so straight-shootingly chic.

- 1953: Marilyn Monroe and Lauren Bacall in *How to Marry a Millionaire*
- 2001: Gwyneth Paltrow in *The Royal Tenenbaums*
- 2006: Meryl Streep in *The Devil Wears Prada*

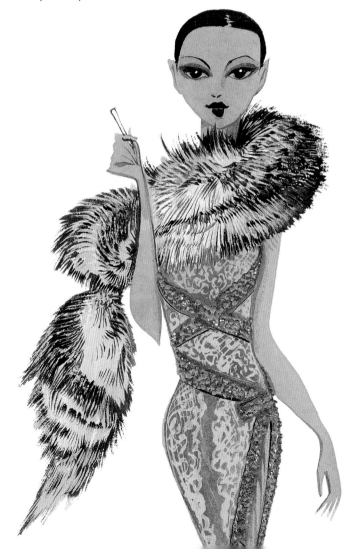

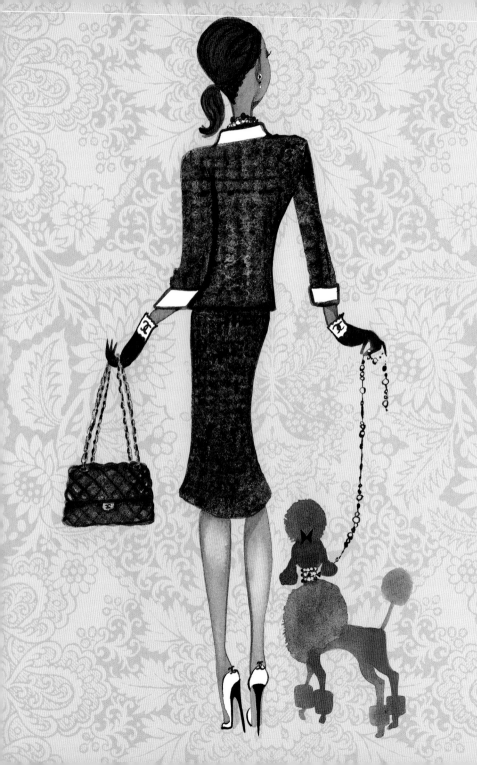

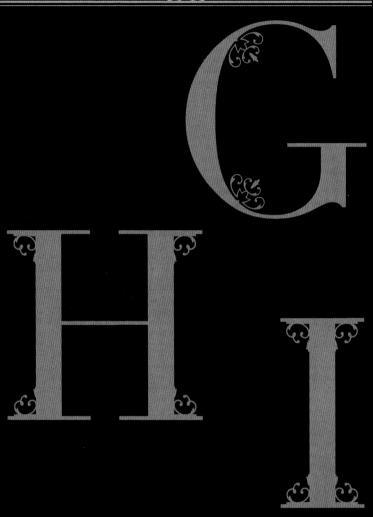

35.
Gentlemen's Hat

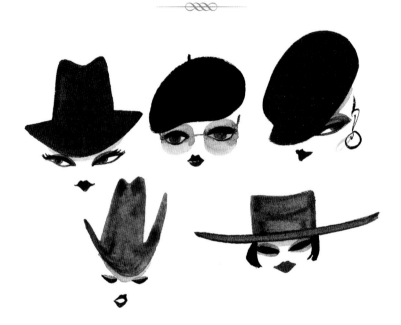

WALKING INTO A ROOM with a man's hat on is much like walking into a room with sunglasses—it will attract and deflect attention at the same time. It will most definitely get you noticed, but you will be able to hide beneath it as well. Every woman should have a gentlemen's hat that she feels comfortable with. There are few things sexier than a woman who just threw one on and walked out to greet the world.

- THE FEDORA: A felt hat creased lengthwise down the crown and pinched on both sides. The fedora is often associated with gangsters and detectives, and though it has found its way to high-fashion heads, it still carries the illusion of menace and mystery. So wear it with attitude. Lots of attitude.
FAMOUS FANS: Greta Garbo, Madonna, Keira Knightley, Frank Sinatra, Al Capone

- TRILBY: Similar to the fedora, but with a narrower brim. The trilby has always been popular among jazz and soul musicians. It has recently gained a following among the indie and emo kids in the UK.
FAMOUS FANS: Agyness Deyn, Justin Timberlake, Victoria Beckham

- THE PANAMA: It is made of plaited toquilla straw and usually has a broad brim and a dented crown. It is light as a feather and has the great advantage of not losing its shape after you roll it up, which makes it perfect for traveling. In an early twentieth-century movie, if it was summertime and the actor was meant to look elegant, you can be sure that the costume director put him in a Panama hat.
FAMOUS FANS: Bob Dylan, Clark Gable

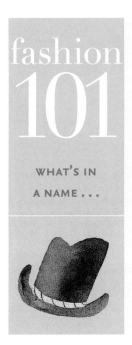

Fedora: Though the fedora is often associated with men, it gets its name from the female character who wore the hat in an 1880s play, *Fedora*.

Trilby: This hat's name also derives from a play, based on the 1894 novel *Trilby*. A hat of this style was worn in the play in the first London production and the name stuck.

Panama: The Panama hat is made in Ecuador, but when the Panama Canal was built, thousands of hats were imported from Ecuador for the construction workers to wear. In 1904, U.S. president Theodore Roosevelt returned from an official visit to the canal wearing one of the hats, and they were forever after known as Panama hats.

THE HAT TRICK

Commit to it. If you don't wear it with confidence, it takes away all the cachet.

Cock your hat—angles are attitudes.

FRANK SINATRA

36.

Gloves

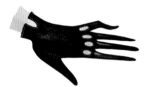

A LONG SATIN OPERA GLOVE conjures images of old Hollywood glamour like nothing else. Think Ava Gardner, Rita Hayworth, Vivien Leigh. All were rarely photographed without wearing gloves. There was a time when no self-respecting actress would be seen without her gloves. Gloves were a symbol of elegance and femininity. Gloves went out of mainstream vogue in the '60s and '70s, when women resisted any of the then-perceived shackles of femininity. And, let's be honest, the long satin opera glove has not exactly made a roaring comeback. But when you see a woman wearing chic, situation-appropriate gloves, it's still very, very glamorous.

FUN FACT

The first opera gloves were worn in 1566 by Queen Elizabeth I, who wore an eighteen-inch pair of white leather gauntlets with gold trim to a ceremony at Oxford.

GLOVE LOVE

- It is important that they fit perfectly—especially at the fingers.
- Wear them with three-quarter length jackets for a safer option.
- If you just can't do the long satin glove, go for an edgy leather driving glove or fingerless version (quite the opposite of Hollywood glamour, but perfect for those days when you feel like playing the badass).

GREAT MOMENTS IN GLOVES

- 1946: Rita Hayworth in *Gilda*
- 1952: Lana Turner in *The Merry Widow*
- 1953: Marilyn Monroe in *Gentlemen Prefer Blondes*
- 1961: Audrey Hepburn in *Breakfast at Tiffany's*
- 1962: Natalie Wood in *Gypsy*

You must have gloves or I won't go.
Gloves are more important than anything else.

MEG IN *LITTLE WOMEN*

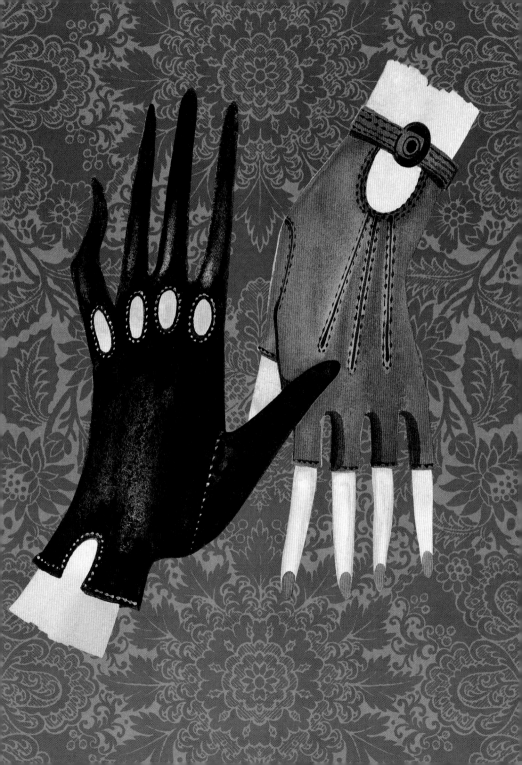

37.

Havaianas

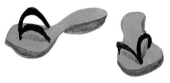

I
N BRAZIL, Havaianas (pronounced *ah-vai-YAH-nas*) are a
national treasure. They are so essential that they are sold in
the supermarket right along with rice and beans. They are
called "the democratic sandal," since everyone from the
average citizen to the highest dignitary wears them. So in
2002, when Jean Paul Gaultier sent fifty models down the runway
in Havaianas, Brazilians were not nearly as intrigued as the rest of
us were. What was it about these flip-flops that made them runway
worthy, we wanted to know. And why was every celebrity suddenly
sporting a pair? And then we tried them on. And we loved them. I
love them.

Sure, they are cute, but the great appeal of the Havaianas is how
butter-soft they are. As soon as you put them on, you are not going to
want to take them off. You realize what the obsession is all about, and
you start justifying wearing flip-flops with just about anything.

*Happiness is owning an old pair of blue jeans
and a new pair of Havaianas.*

ANONYMOUS

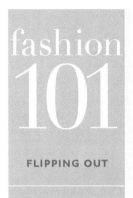

fashion
101

FLIPPING OUT

The original Havaianas (meaning "Hawaiians" in Portuguese) were inspired by the Zori, a Japanese straw sandal originally worn with kimonos. In 1962, shoemaker São Paulo Alpargatas took this idea and decided to make a rubber version, which would suit Brazil's climate better. In 2002, the company finally began exporting the sandals (though tourists had long been smuggling them out of Brazil in their suitcases and selling them in European boutiques).

FUN FACT

If all the Havaianas in the world were laid out end to end, they would go around the world fifty times.

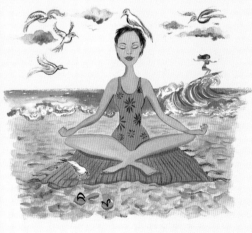

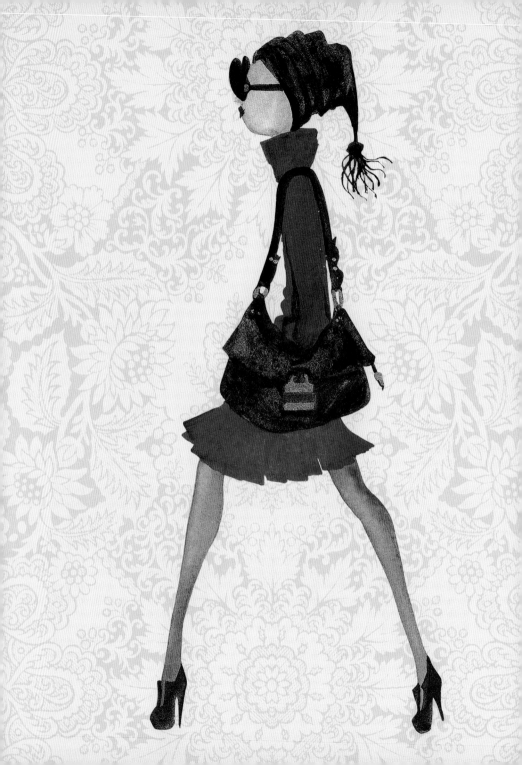

38

Hobo Bag

※

THIS IS the perfect everyday bag because it is spacious (holds all of your essentials), sublimely slouchy (easily slings over your shoulder), and durable (can handle being beat up a bit). The hobo bag was modeled after the large cloth satchels that the hobos used to carry and is often the bag of choice for the bohemian chick, as it is casual and low-key. The hobo bag can be a downtown bag for the artists, models, young "It" girls. But uptown women have a version, too (see the Jackie O bag under Investment Bag, #40), because they realize that the hobo is the ideal everyday bag.

WHERE TO FIND?

Almost every bag line offers a hobo, but a few of my favorites include:

- For the more refined uptown version: Gucci, Coach, Jimmy Choo.
- For the more rugged downtown version: Check Marc by Marc Jacobs if you want to invest. Or go to Anthropologie or Urban Outfitters, where you will find them in cloth, which most resembles the original hobos.

39.
Hoop Earrings

A̲N OLD STANDBY for day or evening. Like the diamond stud, they do not have to be real to do the job. They can be bought at any price point and in an array of styles and sizes. But stick with silver or gold. In general, the thinner, the better. There is a complete correlation between thin and big and thick and short. The bigger and more refined a gold hoop is, the sexier and younger it looks. The smaller and chunkier, the more classic and sophisticated it becomes. And big chunky doorknockers are a definite NO. Unless you're a backup dancer.

HOOP SHOT

- Choose your hoops in proportion to your face, your hair, your neckline.
- The larger and the thinner are the more sexy option.

- Dean Harris hoops: These are the Rolls-Royce of hoop earrings. They are thin but refined. The most beautiful hoops that every fashion editor lusts after.
- XIV Karats: A store in Beverly Hills that carries hoops in gold or silver in every size imaginable. If you want to be fashion-editor neurotic about the width of your hoops, this is the place for you.
- Jacob the Jeweler: The best pavé diamond versions. Again, the thinner, the better.

You can always tell what kind of person a man thinks you are by the earrings he gives you.

AUDREY HEPBURN

40.

Investment Bag

⟨∙∙∙∙∙∙⟩

THIS IS THE BAG that you can spend a few weeks' salary on and not feel guilty (or you *shouldn't*, anyway). It is going to last you a lifetime, will never go out of style, and will only get better with age. It is the bag that is just as relevant today as it was when it debuted fifty or so years ago. And when your granddaughter happens upon it fifty years from now, she will try to steal it. When you are ready and able to spend some big bucks on a big bag, I always say that there are only a handful that are worth your money.

1. The Chanel 2.55
2. LV Speedy
3. The Jackie O
4. The Birkin

Once you recognize them, you realize that every other bag is really a variation on these four. Here is the rundown.

CHANEL 2.55

Coco Chanel's iconic quilted bag, with a double-chain shoulder strap and interlocking Cs as the clasp. When you go in search of your 2.55, the inclination may be to get the plain black calfskin. But because the piece is so classic, don't shy away from some of the wacky styles and colors.

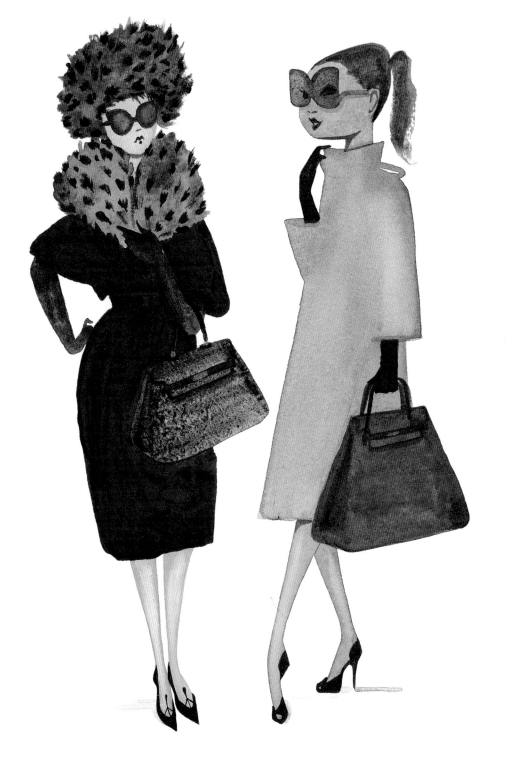

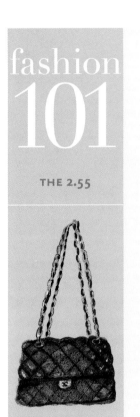

fashion
101

THE 2.55

Coco Chanel's iconic bag was launched in February of 1955, hence the moniker, 2.55. Each feature of the bag—from the lining to the shoulder strap—reveals a bit about Mme Chanel. The brown lining is the color of the uniforms from the convent where she grew up. The inside zippered compartment on the front flap is where she hid her love letters. The back outside flap is where she stashed extra money. The shoulder straps, which were quite uncommon on luxury items at the time, are there because Mme Chanel saw nothing unfeminine about having her hands free.

A girl should be two things: classy and fabulous.

COCO CHANEL

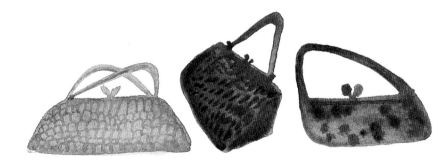

LV SPEEDY BAG

The Louis Vuitton Speedy has been around since 1933 and remains Louis Vuitton's most iconic bag. It is often referred to as the doctor's bag or the doctor's satchel for its resemblance to an old doctor's bag. The classic version has the interlocking LV monogram, but it can also be found in plain leather or with a checkerboard pattern. It is available in three sizes: the Speedy 25 (10" × 7"), the Speedy 30 (12" × 8"), and the Speedy 35 (14" × 9"). The Speedy 30 is by far the most popular.

HOW TO SPOT A FAKE

Louis Vuitton products remain some of the most counterfeited items, so when buying secondhand you have to be very leery. On a real Louis, the LVs are never cut off, the colors are rich, and the hardware is heavy. Mostly you can tell the real from the fake by just looking at the quality of the leather . . . or if you've just paid a serious amount at the Louis Vuitton boutique.

GUCCI JACKIE O BAG

It was Jackie O who made the hobo bag famous, as she carried the double-strapped version everywhere. Women flooded into the Gucci stores and badgered the salesclerks for "the bag that Jackie O always wears," which prompted the company to dub the bag the "Jackie O." It is now known as "the Bouvier" and remains a solid investment. As with the 2.55, don't shy away from the out-of-the-ordinary colors, metallics, and prints that this bag comes in today.

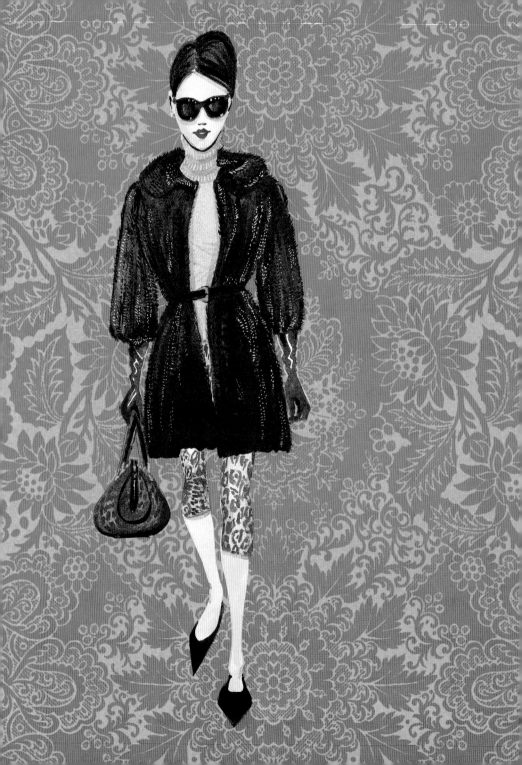

HERMÈS BIRKIN BAG

The Birkin, the rather large, rather expensive tote bag, has reached iconic status. It makes it into song lyrics and TV show scripts, and everyone knows it by name. Because of its massive desirability, there is a two-year waiting list for the bag, causing some to go to extremes to get their hands on it.

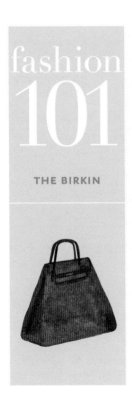

fashion
101

THE BIRKIN

During a 1981 airplane flight, Jane Birkin's over-stuffed purse spilled out into the vicinity of Jean-Louis Dumas-Hermès, which gave Mr. Dumas-Hermès an idea. Three years later, Hermès introduced a bag that was based on an 1892 design. It was large and meant to accommodate Jane Birkin's modern lifestyle. In a wonderful bit of irony, Birkin confessed that she stopped using hers, for she felt it was hazardous to her health.

I told Hermès they were mad to make it.
My one was always full,
and it ended up giving me tendonitis.

JANE BIRKIN

41.
iPod

WHAT STARTED OUT as a utilitarian device is now an essential fashion item. Those recognizable white earbuds have become a ubiquitous accessory on subways and schoolyards the world over (making us all really wish we had bought stock in Apple—how much larger our shoe funds would be!). Each time a new, smaller version comes out, everyone rushes to snag the sleeker model. Some will go so far as to cover them in Swarovski crystals and designer iPod cases. This is fine, but an iPod speaks for itself. And whatever you're listening to, it better be grand.

THE TRULY FASHION OBSESSED HAVE A PLAYLIST THAT GOES A LITTLE SOMETHING LIKE THIS . . .

- "Fashion," David Bowie
- "Supermodel (You Better Work)," RuPaul
- "I'm Too Sexy," Right Said Fred
- "Dress You Up," Madonna
- "Glamorous," Fergie
- "Rich Girl," Gwen Stefani with Eve
- "Girls in Their Summer Clothes," Bruce Springsteen
- "Blue Jean Baby," Elton John
- "Leather Jackets," Elton John

- "She's a Rainbow," Rolling Stones
- "Girl in a T-Shirt," ZZ Top
- "Lady in Red," Chris de Burgh
- "Sunglasses at Night," Corey Hart
- "Imelda," Mark Knopfler
- "Raspberry Beret," Prince
- "Diamonds on the Soles of Her Shoes," Paul Simon
- "New Shoes," Paolo Nutini
- "You Look Good in My Shirt," Keith Urban
- "Addicted to Love," Robert Palmer (the video version)
- "Freedom," George Michael (the video version)

*After silence, that which comes nearest
to expressing the inexpressible is music.*

ALDOUS HUXLEY

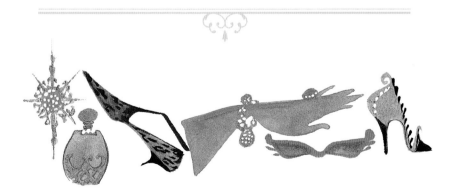

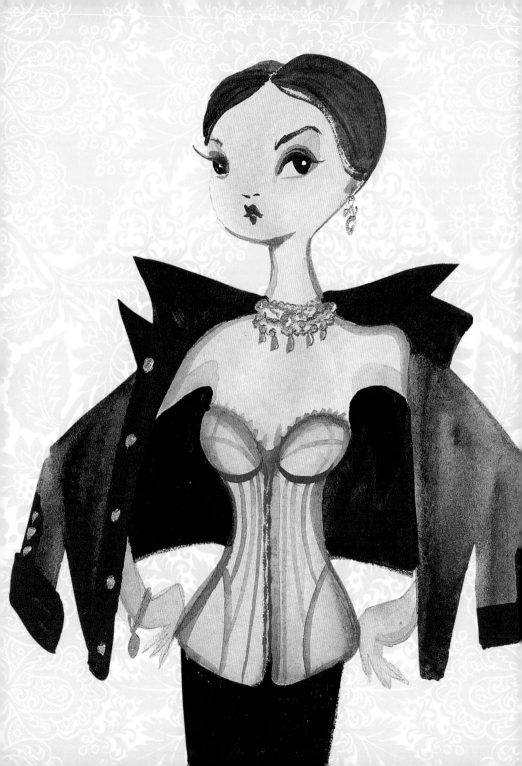

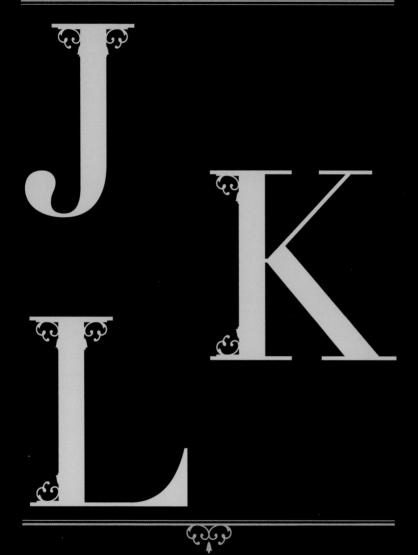

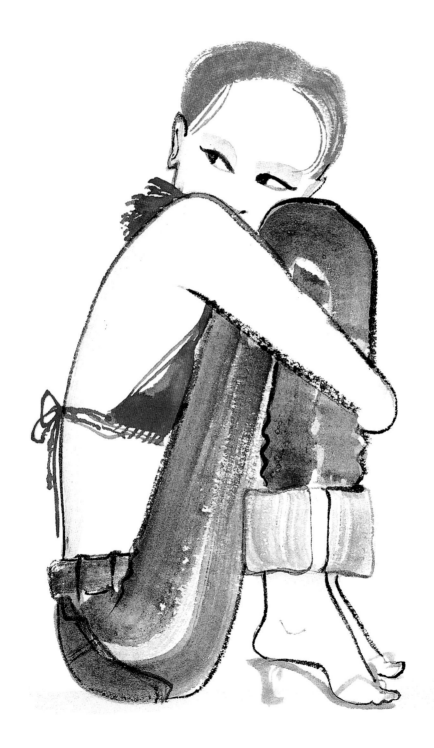

42.

Jeans

————⌀⌀⌀————

I AM ALWAYS ASKED, "What is the best jean?" I panic every time. It changes every damn day and I always think, "Why don't I know this?" I don't know because there is a denim snobbism that has taken over our simple blue jeans. "Who are you wearing? Oh, you can't wear those anymore! You have to buy [insert jean of the week here]." The irony of it is laughable. One of the most simple, most casual items in the world has turned into such a headache for women. We need a Zagat's to navigate it all. Don't let any of this get to you. Pick a jean that fits you perfectly and stick with it, no matter the brand. Fit is everything, and the very nature of denim is that it's so democratic. Be you and the jean will, too.

Blue jeans are the most beautiful thing
since the gondola.

DIANA VREELAND

THE SKINNY: FOUR TYPES OF JEAN BUYERS

- **The Classicist:** She buys 501s, Lees, or Wranglers. She is known to sift through vintage stores that have pairs that are worn in already, and when she puts them on, they look like they have been hers for twenty years. She could not care less what the jean of the moment is.
- **The Fashion Follower:** She follows jeans like the stock market. If you want to know what the "the" brand is, she knows. She will tell you exactly how the pockets should be, who the "It" brand was last week, and who it may be next week (Earnest Sewn, True Religion, Diesel).
- **The Euro:** She wears only the designer jeans (Gucci, Prada, Versace).
- **The Eco:** She wears only environmentally friendly jeans like Rogan and Edun.

I do not know when the continental rift occurred, but I do know that is has become very stressful to buy jeans. It is very stressful, that is, until you realize that it's not the label or the cost that makes a pair of jeans perfect; it's the way they fit and the way they make you feel. Mostly, it's about how you look when you walk away . . .

BLUE JEAN BABY

We've all been there. Standing in the dressing room, pulling, trying on a tenth pair of jeans as the salesgirl calls, "How you making out?" You just want to reach out and strangle her. But instead you calm yourself, peek out, and ask if she might be able to bring you a few more in your size. And the size below your size. And the size above. But then, on the twentieth or thirtieth try, you find them. Your perfect match. Sure, they'll need a little altering and a bit of breaking in, but for the most part, it will be love at first sight.

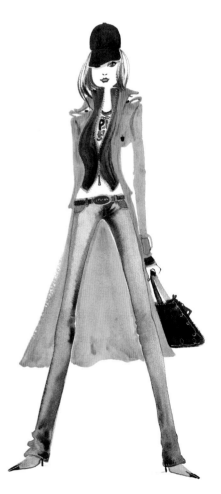

- Do not assume that because a brand is expensive or a friend or celebrity "swears by them" that they will be the right jeans for you. One brand does not suit all.
- Try a jean with stretch. A revelation and a revolution.
- Consider a white jean or a black jean.
- Expect to have them tailored. It's rare to find a pair of jeans that fit you right off the rack.
- Try out every brand, style, size. Seek and ye shall find.

fashion 101

DENIM, DECADE BY DECADE

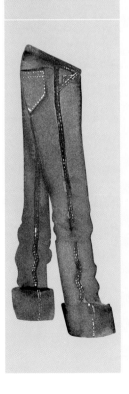

- **1853:** The California Gold Rush. The gold miners wanted strong, sturdy clothes, and Leo Strauss (who later changed his name to Levi) started a wholesale business to meet the demand.
- **1930s:** Jeans gained notoriety when actors started to wear them in all the popular Western movies.
- **1940s:** American soldiers introduced jeans to the world when they wore them while they were off duty.
- **1950s:** Denim became a symbol of teenage rebellion (think James Dean in *Rebel Without a Cause*), and jeans became immensely popular among the young, so much so that some schools in the United States banned students from wearing them.
- **1960s–70s:** Jeans were made to match the hippie fashions (painted, embroidered, flared, psychedelic, etc.).
- **1980s:** Denim went high fashion and famous designers started to make their own jean designs with their labels.
- **1990s:** Sales went on the decline as teenagers turned to khakis, combat, and carpenter pants. If they *did* opt for jeans, they went for vintage pairs found in secondhand stores. Eleven North American Levi Strauss factories closed.
- **2000s:** Jeans came back with a vengeance, appearing on every runway, on every store floor, in every fashion magazine. Now there are innumerable brands to choose from, and somehow, the humble jean has become a sort of status symbol.

43

Jewelry Pouches

THESE ARE VITAL ACCESSORIES when traveling. You should have several velvet or silk pouches so none of your pieces of jewelry gets lost, chipped, or tangled. They are available at any jewelry store, but you can also use the luxe bags that high-end alcohol comes in. For decades, girls have been asking the bartender for the velvety purple Crown Royal bags. You won't be the first. Also useful for storing shoes, sunglasses, and spare change.

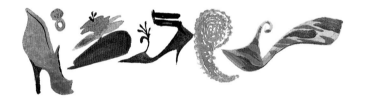

Jewelry takes people's minds off your wrinkles.

SONJA HENIE

44.
Khakis

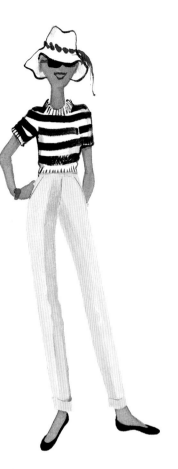

THE TAN cotton twill fabric will forever be associated with prep schools and polo matches, but is also found on the runways every season. They can be high fashion (think khaki jodhpurs paired with schoolboy blazers) or low-key (rumpled chinos and a white Hanes T-shirt à la Diane Keaton in *Annie Hall*). It's often the pant of choice for casual girls who want to kick it up just a notch from the standard jeans.

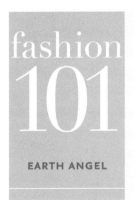

fashion 101

EARTH ANGEL

Khaki, the Hindi-Urdu word for *earth-colored*, was invented in nineteenth-century India. The British Army wanted to save their white uniforms from the windblown dust, so they began dyeing their clothes in coffee and curry powder. The fabric became the standard for British and American army uniforms and later became a favorite among the upper-class and preppy.

45.
Knee Boots

U NTIL THE 1960S, boots were men's territory. Women wore them in times of inclement weather, but never as fashion objects. Then, in the 1960s, when Mary Quant introduced the miniskirt, André Courrèges met her with the boot, and legs took center stage. It started at midcalf and was dubbed the "go-go boot" because it was ideal for dancing. As skirts got shorter, boots got higher (sometimes going up to the thigh) and truly became a sign of female liberation. The boot has maintained its appeal and remains a sign of sexuality and power; it is still quite useful for making men go weak at the knees.

HIGH POINTS FOR HIGH BOOTS

ON SCREEN
- 1968: Jane Fonda in *Barbarella*
- 1997: Heather Graham in *Austin Powers*
- All of Charlie's Angels

IN SONG
- "These Boots Are Made for Walking," Nancy Sinatra
- "Kinky Boots," Patrick Macnee and Honor Blackman
- "Don't Go Away Go Go Girl," The Mr. T Experience

BOOT UP

- The version that every girl needs comes just below the knee and looks best when worn with skirts that hit just above the knee.
- If you want to be daring, get the boot that goes above the knee, or if you want to be a bit mod, get one that hits mid-calf (the go-go boot).
- If wearing knee-high boots with miniskirts, it's probably best to wear opaque tights.

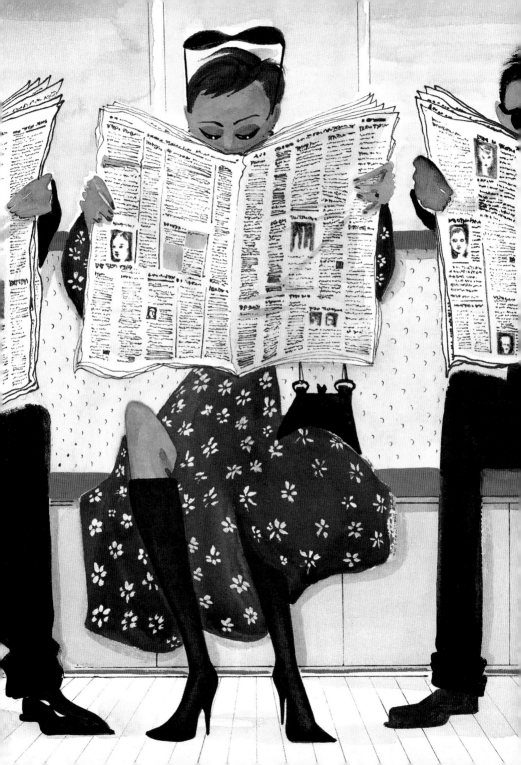

46.
Leather Pants

WEARING LEATHER PANTS means something. It's primal, it's sexual (it is skin-on-skin, after all), and it means you are ready to rock 'n' roll and/or break a few hearts. They must be worn with confidence and badass attitude. Think Mick Jagger on stage singing about how he couldn't get no satisfaction (which I never quite believe), or Lenny Kravitz singing about an American woman who won't let him be (which I definitely believe). Think Joan Jett, Debbie Harry, Madonna, Janis Joplin. They all wore 'em and they wore 'em well, with kick-ass confidence and a badass attitude. Leather pants are an article of clothing for the tough, confident, sexy rock star. There's a little rocker chick in all of us, so we'd best have the leather pants for those days she feels like breaking out.

THE COOL KIDS TO COPY

· Jim Morrison
· Mick Jagger
· Lenny Kravitz
· Angelina Jolie
· Joan Jett
· Catwoman

- Chrome Hearts: The couture of leather pants.
- Lost Art: Custom-made leather. This is the company that makes Lenny Kravitz's pants.

ROCKING OUT

- Find a pair that is form-fitting. Try a size down from your usual, since the leather will stretch a bit.
- But be sure not to go too tight. You want to show off your curves, not cut off your circulation.
- Keep it simple. Any additions like laces up the sides or studs will drastically deplete the cool factor.
- Do not wear your leather pants with your leather jacket... unless you plan on being on the back of a motorcycle all afternoon.

I love rock 'n' roll, so put another dime
in the jukebox, baby . . .

JOAN JETT & THE BLACKHEARTS

47.
Lingerie

~~~

INGERIE IS ABOUT more than just bras (see Push-Up Bra, #70) and thongs (see Underwear, #90). Every woman needs a few other essential undergarments for practical reasons, but also for personal reasons. Sometimes it's what you put on before you get dressed that makes the outfit. Sometimes it's just to make you feel sexy and boost your confidence (a silk slip to sleep in), and other times it's to serve a function (a silk slip to wear under your dress).

I know some women who have entire drawers devoted to their impressive lingerie collections. But when it comes right down to it, here are the big four necessities:

- CAMISOLE: To go under all the blazers and jackets on this list.
- SILK SLIP: To go under those dresses that are questionably thin or too clingy.
- NEGLIGEE: To sleep in and feel amazingly sexy when you need something a notch up from your standard pajamas (see Pajamas, #62).
- SILK STOCKINGS: To drive men wild. Forget sex toys, these are all you need.

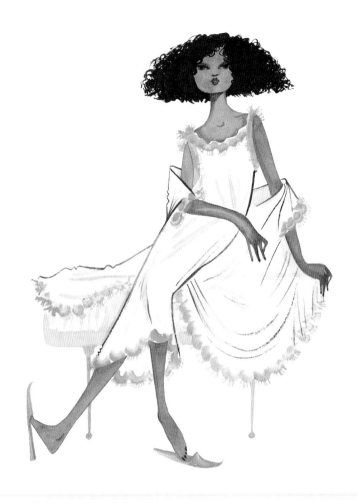

*If you're wearing lingerie
that makes you feel glamorous,
you're halfway there to turning heads.*

ELLE MACPHERSON

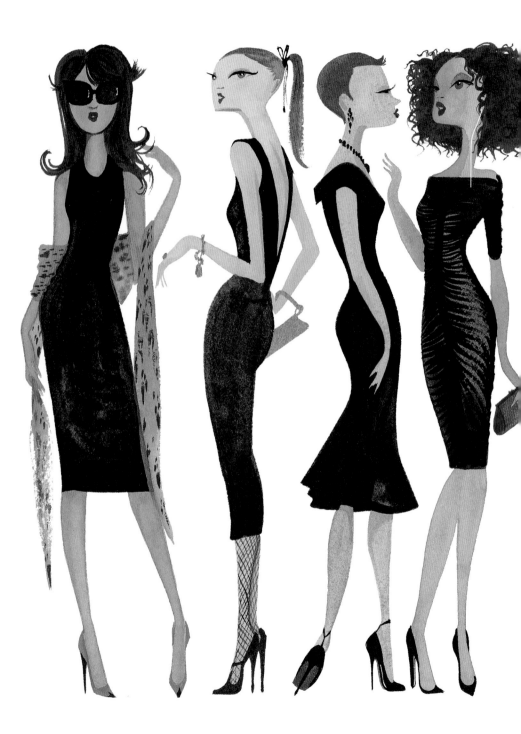

48.

Little Black Dress

⎯⎯⎯⎯ ⧜ ⎯⎯⎯⎯

OFTEN, the perfect little black dress finds a girl when she is not looking. If she sets out on a "perfect little black dress mission," the thing will elude her all afternoon. But if she is on her way to a lazy Sunday brunch, it will most likely jump out at her from the storefront window. No matter what the cost, she should buy it. It may be H&M or it may be Alaia. The price is immaterial, since it can always be justified by the rules of fashion math: cost divided by number of times worn equals priceless. It will be there time after time, decade after decade.

BACK IN BLACK

- Choose the best material you can find (not all are created equal) and nothing too tight or too shiny.
- Consider your LBD a blank canvas instead of a fallback. It demands to be accessorized and adorned.
- To avoid being accused of playing it safe, make sure you have a dash of daring (a dangerous stiletto, bold jewelry, etc.), and make sure it shows off your best assets.
- Remember, the reason the simple garment is so enduring

is because it understands the essence of style: to step back and let the woman shine. So shine.

- It is said that you need only one, but a minimum of two is a better guideline.
- Make sure you can dance in it.

fashion
101

THE LITTLE
BLACK DRESS

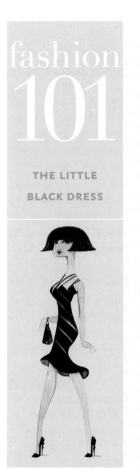

As mentioned in my first book, *The Little Black Book of Style*, fashion history credits Coco Chanel with inventing the little black dress in 1926. Yet women had been wearing little black dresses long before. It should be noted, however, that it wasn't until the 1920s that the black dress became a fashion statement, and not a dress simply for practicality or mourning. And for that, we must give it up to Mme Chanel. She would insist on it, in fact. She might say that she knew about the power of the black dress before anyone else, and she might be right. When Paul Poiret came up to her in one of her first little black creations, he asked, "For whom, Madame, do you mourn?" She cheekily responded, "For you, Monsieur." Turns out, she knew what she was talking about.

And we should also give it up to Mme Chanel for coming up with the moniker of "little black dress" while she was criticizing her fashion rival Elsa Schiaparelli. "Scheherazade is easy," she noted. "The little black dress is hard."

Clearly, Mme Chanel was not a woman to mess with, which is why, after much reflection and research, I'm going to give her a little credit here. Yes, the little black dress has been in existence for centuries, but where it was once an item of practicality and solemnity, it is now a sure sign of power and sensuality. And for that, we can thank Mme Chanel.

- 1961: Audrey Hepburn (does it even bear repeating?) wears the famed Givenchy LBD in *Breakfast at Tiffany's.*
- 1972: The Hollies debut their hit "Long Cool Woman in a Black Dress." *That long cool woman had it all. . .*
- 1986: Robert Palmer's "Addicted to Love" video airs on MTV, showcasing top models in little black dresses. The world—especially the fashion world—drools.
- 1986: Cher attends the Oscars in an awe/shock-inspiring Bob Mackie number. ("As you can see, I did receive my Academy booklet on how to dress like a serious actress.") This little black dress went a long way, showing how diverse a concept the LBD can be.
- 1994: Elizabeth Hurley goes to the *Four Weddings and a Funeral* premiere in a little black dress by Versace, held together with safety pins. Her career skyrockets.
- 1994: Princess Diana steps out in that memorable black dress the night Prince Charles made that memorable announcement.
- 1996: U2 debuts the song "Little Black Dress," lyrically praising the power of the item. *Here she comes like a child with a gun . . .*
- 2006: The LBD from *Breakfast at Tiffany's* is sold at auction for £467,000 (roughly $920,909).

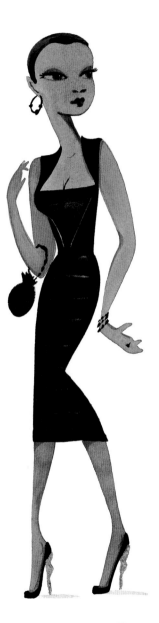

When the little black dress is right,
there is nothing else to wear in its place.

WALLIS SIMPSON, DUCHESS OF WINDSOR

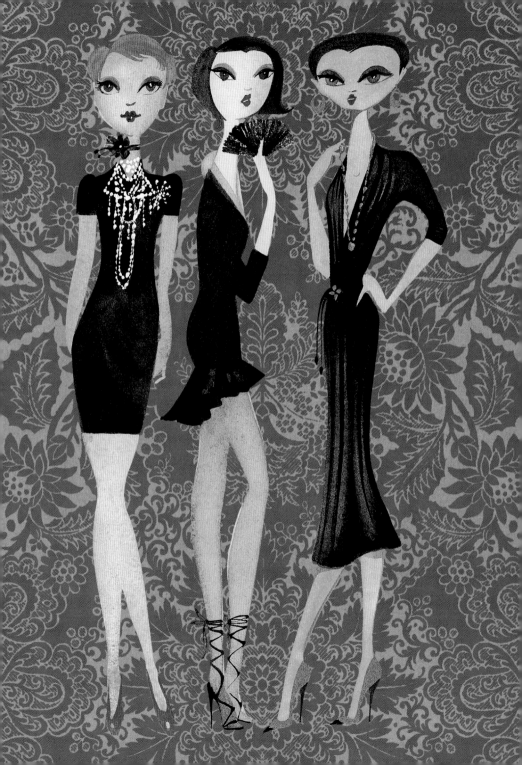

49.
Little White Dress

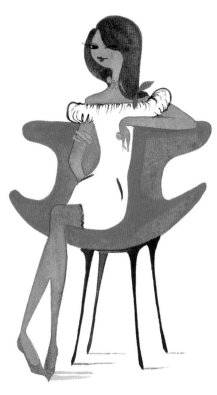

THE LITTLE WHITE DRESS does not get nearly as much love as the LBD, and it's a pity. Everyone needs a little white dress. After all, what else would a girl wear when returning from vacation to show off her tan and provoke the jealous? The LWD is the unsung hero of the dress department. And it is by far the best dress to wear to usher in summer and to wear in the winter to show that you've never followed a "no white after Labor Day" kind of rule in your life. Though it is advisable not to order red sauce or red wines when wearing the pure white dress. An accident while wearing white is not an accident, but a tragic disaster.

WHITE NIGHTS

- Try a shoe in gold, silver, or nude with the little white dress.
- Shake all associations with innocence and purity by wearing edgy jewelry (a gold snake choker, an unexpected armband, or an obnoxiously large cocktail ring).

A white dress she had on.
She was carrying a white parasol.
I only saw her for one second. She didn't see me at all.
But I'll bet a month hasn't gone by
since that I hadn't thought of that girl.

CITIZEN KANE

50.
L.L.Bean Tote

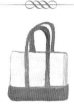

A CENTURY AGO, a lady did not carry a bag larger than a clutch (and a small clutch at that). Today, we carry our lives around on our shoulders, making weekly massages quite justifiable and an L.L.Bean bag a necessity. The L.L.Bean tote is, as the company states, "the toughest tote you can buy." Nothing is too heavy for this bag—believe me, I've given it a run for its money. It was originally created in the '40s, and was meant for carrying ice and firewood. I can attest that it also works quite well for toting: several bottles of wine to the park; a summer reading list's worth of books; a beach day's worth of snacks, sunscreen, and sand toys; twenty-seven fashion magazines (double issues included); a laptop and hundreds of dog-eared manuscript pages, and on and on.

FUN FACT

The classic L.L.Bean tote was introduced in 1944 as Bean's Ice Carrier.

- I recommend having several of these around the house. You will always find uses for them.
- Get them monogrammed!
- It is available in four sizes. The large is the most popular and, in my opinion, the best one.
- There is an extra-large version, which seems too large for everyday use. But if you need to carry a lot of firewood, ice, or wine, perhaps it is your best bet.
- If you want to go high-end, get a textured leather so the scratches don't show too much. Make sure the lining is durable (leather or suede), that there are studs/feet on the bottom to protect it as much as possible, and that the shoulder straps are comfortable.

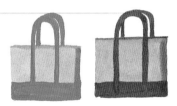

In character, in manner, in style, in all things, the supreme excellence is simplicity.

HENRY WADSWORTH LONGFELLOW

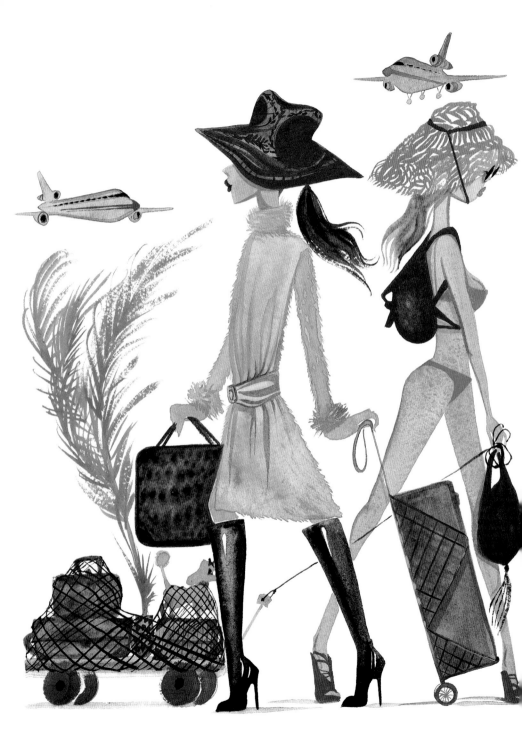

51.
Luggage

⎯⎯⎯⎯⎯ ∞∞∞ ⎯⎯⎯⎯⎯

THE LUCKY CAN BUY an entire matching set at once, but otherwise it is best to buy one piece at a time, starting with a small carry-on roller (which ensures that you cannot overpack) and building up to a large suitcase (which ensures that you *will* overpack). The matching duffel is also an essential piece since it can be used as an overnight/weekend bag or a carry-on.

FASHION EDITOR FAVORITES

- Kate Spade, Coach: **Both really adorable, colorful.**
- Samsonite, Tumi: **Durable and dependable.**
- Globe-Trotter: **A very cool company out of England. Strictly for rock stars who are willing to spend money for custom-made luggage.**
- T. Anthony LTD: **A luxury brand known for its mono-grammed pieces. The Windsors' favorite (they owned 118 trunks).**
- Ghurka: **Perfect if you feel like going on safari (or need a good gift for outdoorsman boyfriend).**
- Longchamp: **Great luggage. Also make totes that fold into**

little envelopes—they are perfect for fitting in your luggage on the way there and filling with your purchases on the way back.
- Goyard: The luxury trunkmaker's bags are expensive and hard to get your hands on (available at only a few shops worldwide), but if you can afford it, Goyard is the luggage.
- Louis Vuitton: The clear fashionista favorite. They only look better as they age!
- Private labels: Department store labels—Barneys, for example—are often a good way to get great-looking luggage without spending a ton of money.
- Generic black nylon: Again, if you don't want to spend a ton, get generic black nylon bags, and personalize them with vacation beads and stickers.

BAGGAGE CLAIM

- Get it monogrammed so it's easier to find on the baggage carousel.
- Items to always store in your carry-on: a black cashmere turtleneck, underwear, a toothbrush, a bathing suit, cosmetics bag, all jewelry (maybe a bikini, depending on where you are going).

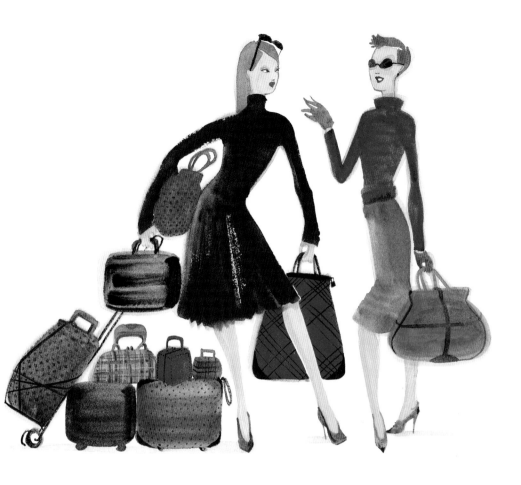

A woman never goes anywhere but the hospital without packing makeup, clothes, and jewelry.

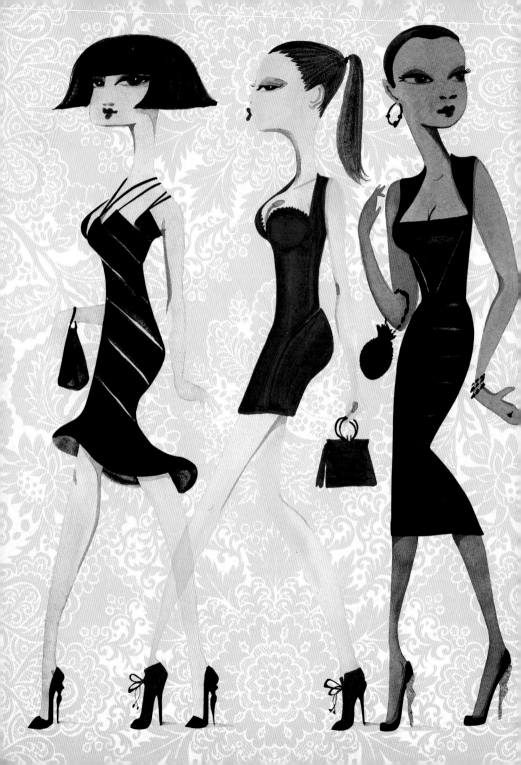

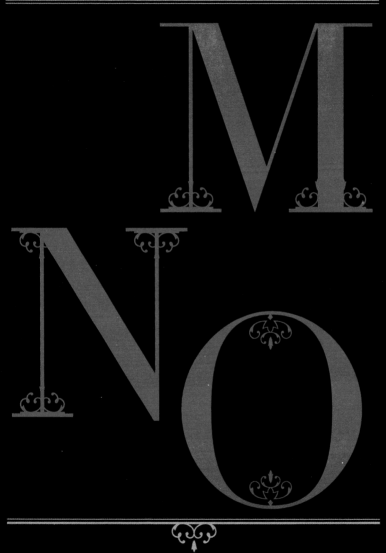

52.
Mad Money

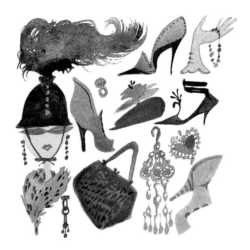

MAD MONEY is the spare fifty-dollar bill you should keep in the secret pocket of your purse or wallet. Place it there and forget about it. You are allowed to spend it only in an emergency, and as soon as you spend it, you must replace it.

The expression "mad money" was coined by Howard J. Savage at the end of an article on slang at Bryn Mawr College. He defined it as "money a girl carries in case she has a row with her escort and wishes to go home alone." I define it as "money a girl carries in case she gets in a fight with her date and wants to go home alone or if she is walking by a vintage shop that doesn't accept credit cards and she finds the perfect little black dress, clutch, or cocktail ring."

53

Man's White Shirt

L IKE the Boyfriend Cardigan (#12), best when stolen out of a husband's closet, though scouring the men's department works well, too. On a man, it is *crisp*, clean, and conservative. But throw it on a woman's body, and the thing sizzles. It quietly whispers suggestions of morning-after dressing, which may or may not be the case, but it does raise the question. And perhaps that is why seeing a woman in a man's white shirt makes women a tad jealous and men more than a tad intrigued. Make sure it's a real men's shirt, though (or close to it). The tapered, tailored, semifitted women's versions take away the cachet and are not quite as chic.

WHO'S GOT IT? EVERYONE . . .

- BROOKS BROTHERS: The best noniron version out there.
- GAP: As classic as they come.
- TARGET: Stock up when they have them in stock.
- Your significant other's closet.

WHITE HOT

- Keep it as close to a man's version as possible.
- No pearl buttons, no novelty buttons, no covered buttons.
- The best buttons look like (or are) mother-of-pearl, and are sewn on a thick, double-plated placket. They should be sewn on with cross-stitching.
- Keep it basic. Go classic cotton or fine linen.

- 1953: Audrey Hepburn in *Roman Holiday.*
- 1956: Elizabeth Taylor in *Giant.*
- 1990: Julia Roberts in *Pretty Woman.*
- 1994: Uma Thurman in *Pulp Fiction.*
- 1998: Sharon Stone on the red carpet at the 70th Annual Academy Awards.

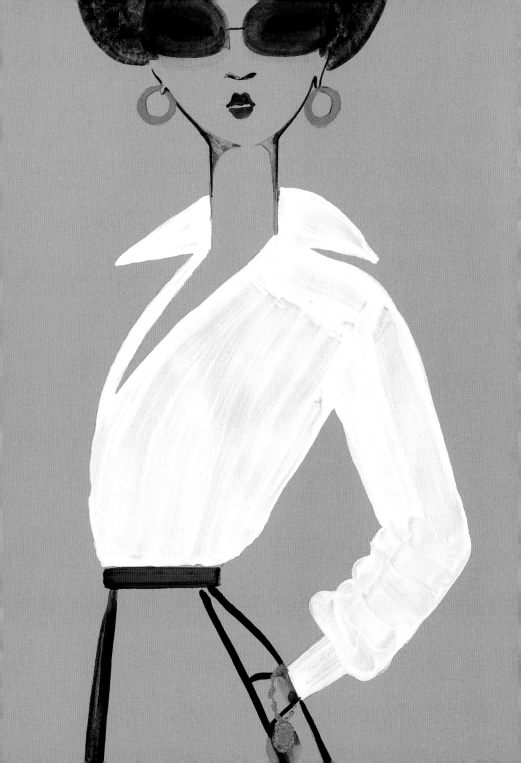

54.

Mary Janes

HERE IS A LOLITA FACTOR about the mary jane that makes it so utterly desirable. It is, after all, the shoe we all wore as little girls, but when it is given a heel and pointed toe, it becomes something else altogether. It brings out the sweet and the sexy in one fell swoop. It makes admirers coo, "Oh, how adorable," but also "Oh, how amazing."

Every season, there is some lusted-after version of the mary jane. The best are usually done by Manolo Blahnik, Christian Louboutin . . . and Christian Louboutin. Miuccia Prada also always has a version that goes strolling down her runway. But if you want to invest in a mary jane, go for the Manolo Blahnik version with the stiletto heel and the pointed toe. It caused a frenzy when it was first created, became impossible to find, and is still considered *the* mary jane.

FUN FACT

The mary jane became popular in the '20s and '30s, when hemlines rose and there was more of an emphasis on the shoes. Mary janes became a favorite because they looked great *and* you could dance in them, a necessary feature in the '20s.

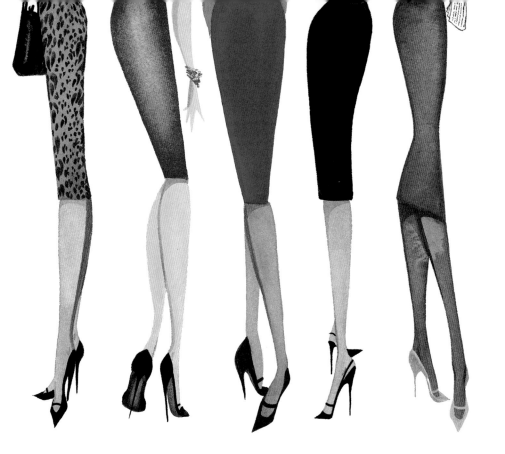

STRAPPED

- It is best in patent, but why not try velvet or an animal print?
- They should have a bit of an edge. A sky-high heel and pointed toe, maybe studs. They cannot be purely sweet and demure.
- It is best if the strap is thin, so it doesn't cut off the leg.

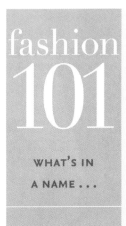

fashion
101

WHAT'S IN
A NAME . . .

The name comes from a comic book character, Mary Jane, who wore strapped shoes in the *Buster Brown* comic strip. Mary Jane's brother, Buster Brown, also had a shoe named after him.

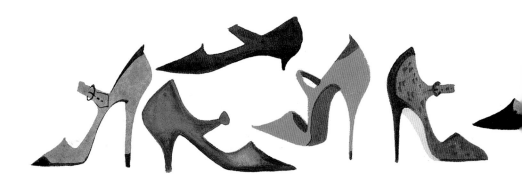

Do you know what these are?
Manolo Blahnik mary janes.
I thought these were an urban shoe myth!

CARRIE BRADSHAW

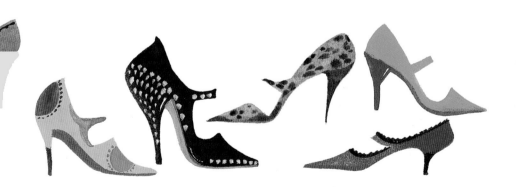

55.
Minnetonka Moccasin

THE MOCCASIN IS sneakily stylish. It will always be a shoe that shows off your free-spirited, relaxed side. They are old-school, low-key, and casual classics. They are great in both the boot and ankle versions, and are incredible when paired with skinny jeans and T-shirts, or cutoff denim shorts and bare legs à la Kate Moss. But never with socks! Generally worn by laid-back girls who want to flaunt that I'm-not-trying-too-hard look that is inherently a part of the moccasin. Many people have made fashion versions of the original, but the original is still the hands-down favorite.

FUN FACT

The design of beads on the front of the moccasin was used to indicate one's tribe.

fashion
101

MINNETONKA
MOCCASIN

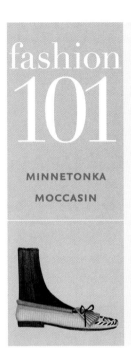

Moccasins, America's first footwear, have been worn by Native Americans for hundreds of years, but they have been worn by city dwellers and suburbanites only since the 1940s. After WWII, when Americans took to the highways, they stopped and shopped at Native American reservations along the way. Many travelers bought pairs of Minnetonkas to bring home, and the Minnetonka moccasin quickly became a casual classic.

Before I judge anyone,
let me first walk a mile in their moccasins.

NATIVE AMERICAN PROVERB

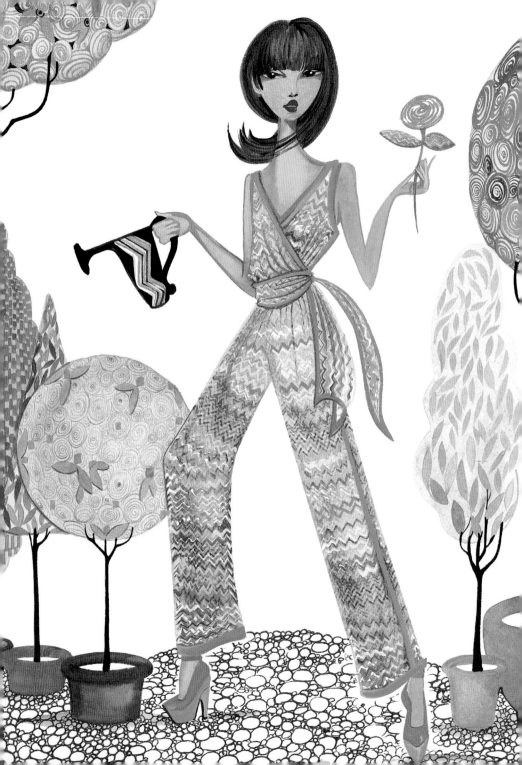

56.
Missoni Knit

WHENEVER A WOMAN steps out in a Missoni, most other women will instantly spot it and envy it from afar. This reaction is pretty much a given. And then they will focus in a little closer to see how many prints and colors and fabrics Missoni managed to fit onto just one incredible garment. It's a thing of beauty, really. There are likely to be stripes mixed with zigzags, cottons mixed with furs. Wools, rayons, linens, and silks. Florals and geometrics. The combinations are endlessly brilliant. Missoni's designs are distinguished by their unique mismatching patterns, prints, and colors. Nothing is off-limits when it comes to a Missoni, and that's exactly why they're known, recognized, and admired the world over.

There are certain designer items that are unmistakable, unforgettable, and unrivaled. There is no substitution and there is also no devaluation of such pieces. A Missoni knit dress definitely meets this criterion. Can you buy other knit dresses? Of course. But will they still be current in ten, twenty, or thirty seasons? It's not likely.

Rosita Missoni states her view of what they create perfectly by saying, "Our philosophy since we went into business has been that a piece of clothing should be like a work of art."

Whenever I wear Missoni, I do feel like a work of art. And all women deserve, at one point when wearing something beautiful, to feel this good.

fashion
101

MISSONI

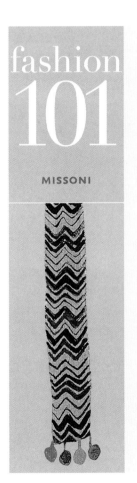

The company was founded by Ottavio ("Tai") Missoni and his wife, Rosita, in 1953, the year they were married. The couple met at the 1948 Olympics. Ottavio had designed the tracksuits for the Italian national team (sidenote: He had been the Italian 400-meter running champion in 1938, and in 1948 he was a finalist in the 400-meter hurdles). Rosita worked at her family's knitwear factory. The two met at Wembley in London, married five years later, and combined forces to create knitwear (Rosita's forte) with crazy and colorful patterns (Tai's brainchild). Their fame was solidified when in 1967 they were invited to show at the Pitti Palace in Florence. At the last minute, Rosita told the models to remove their bras because they showed through the thin blouses. The blouses became transparent under the lights and caused a sensation. The Missonis were not invited back the following year.

Now, over forty years later, the Missoni company is as shock- and awe-inducing as ever. It has never lost its sense of fun, vitality, and youth. Perhaps this is because the family-run business keeps pulling the younger generation of Missonis into the crazy mix. Angela Missoni is now at the helm, and her daughter, Margherita, is one of the most fashionable girls out there, carrying on the name and the Missoni tradition.

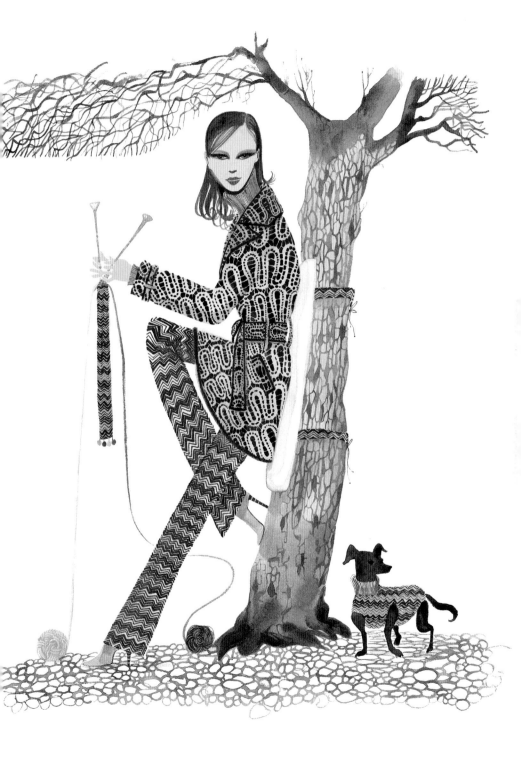

57.
Monogrammed Stationery

WHEN I OPEN an envelope and find within it a note written on monogrammed stationery, I will always put that note on my bulletin board. It's that special to me. In an age of one-line e-mails and three-letter text messages, when an entire generation can say "idk my bff jill" and be understood, a handwritten note is golden. A true class act uses monogrammed stationery. A handwritten note—even the most simple handwritten note—carries so much more meaning than an e-mail.

Don't get me wrong. I am a fan of e-mail. It's the way of the world in which we live. I love to hear the ding of my BlackBerry, only to find an old friend has dropped me a line. But just imagine it: a fully thought-out note, with complete sentences, every word spelled out, and a simple monogram on the top. Is there anything more stylish than that? No, there really isn't.

A FEW OF MY FAVORITE STATIONERS INCLUDE:

- Mrs. John L. Strong: The company was founded in New York in 1929 and is known for making exquisite hand-engraved stationery. Its "ready to write" collection is focused toward a younger, fashionista crowd. I'm a huge fan.
- Crane & Co.: Fine stationery made of 100% cotton, it has been "green" since its beginnings in 1801. Crane's has a wide selection of styles, so you can be as modern or old-fashioned as you'd like. Kate Spade's collections are available from Crane's, which are always dependably simple and stylish.
- Smythson of Bond Street: This luxury company has been the foremost British stationer since the early 1900s. In addition to simple monogrammed stationery, it also produces elaborate bespoke stationery with personalized borders. If you want to be really over-the-top and truly make a statement, this is the way to go.

You don't really know a woman until she writes you a letter.

ADA LEVERSON

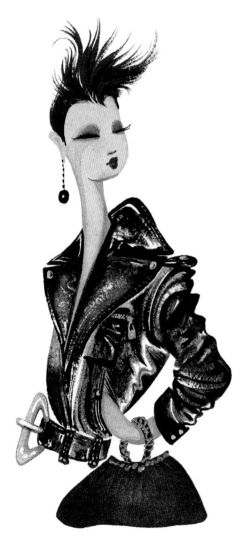

58

Motorcycle Jacket

IT HAS BEEN part of the perennial uniform of cool kids for quite some time now. It is *the* jacket of subcultures: bikers, rock 'n' rollers, punk rockers, metalheads, rebels (with or without a cause). And because the fashion world loves subcultures, the motorcycle jacket will always be the jacket of choice for the absolutely stylish. Every model, actress, and musician has her old faithful version to throw on when she feels the need for that elusive cool factor. It should be in your closet for days when you want to channel Françoise Hardy or Marianne Faithfull or the Sex Pistols. Or all three at once—it definitely communicates a super "It" factor.

REBEL YELL

- To avoid looking like you are stuck in the '80s, stick to black and avoid any shiny, cheap leather. Only the best hides for the motorcycle set. Also, avoid the double-breasted or the crossover. Few can carry these off in a way befitting a style rebel.
- Proportions are key. Either go oversized or shrunken. Steal it from the boys or go down a size. There are no in-betweens.
- Beat up is best. Vintage is great—all of the best leather jackets seem to be hiding in LA vintage shops. (There are a few items that are best found in LA vintage shops, and this is one of them.)
- Wear it with the usual suspects: skinny pants, short skirts, denim, and denim skirts. But also dare to pair it with a feminine dress or a pencil skirt and camisole. For a total French look, wear it with a white sailor top, skinny pants, and flats. But no matter what, keep the jewelry to a minimum. The biker babe and diamonds just don't live in harmony with each other.

- Rick Owens: The new coolest-kid-on-the-block. He has these amazing, paper-thin versions that all the fashion-insiders adore. Owens sums it up best: "I'd describe my work as Frankenstein and Garbo, falling in love in a leather bar."
- Topshop, H&M, Forever 21: All make great inexpensive versions. If we are going on a shoot and need a leather jacket in a pinch, we can always depend on these chains. Rebel on demand.
- Alexander McQueen, Balenciaga, Comme des Garçons, Gucci: These are the standbys and the mainstays. They will always have a good motorcycle jacket in stock, and you can be sure it will be a classic, enduring version. The cost may set you back a bit, but in the end, you've invested in a piece that invokes attitude and sass. Worth every single dollar.

"What're you rebelling against, Johnny?"
"Whaddya got?"

THE WILD ONE,
WHERE MARLON BRANDO MADE THE LEATHER JACKET
THE REBEL UNIFORM

fashion 101

FASHION VS. FUNCTION

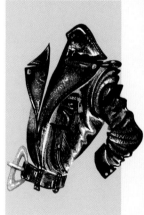

The leather jacket was born out of function and was meant to protect bikers should they hit the concrete. The original, the Schott Perfecto, was created in 1928. At the time, the jacket sold for $5.50 at a Harley-Davidson shop in Long Island. The design was durable, rugged, and immediately embraced by the biking community. It is still sold today (though no longer for $5.50!) and is a great fashion statement in and of itself. However, it is nothing like the Rick Owens and Balenciaga versions we wear today.

On a real motorcycle jacket, each feature is chosen out of practicality. The leather will be at least a millimeter thick to protect riders from the road. There will also be more usable pocket space and better weather protection. The back may be slightly dropped so the rider can comfortably lean forward and keep the wind out. The sleeves are usually precurved. A leather jacket created for fashion has none of these features. The leather is generally much thinner, the pockets are placed more for aesthetics than for storage, the sleeves are not precurved, etc. But, of course, if the leather jacket is made right, it will look cool either way—whether you are biking or hitting the Friday-night club circuit.

59.
Nail Polish

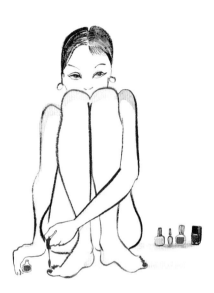

NAIL POLISH should go to extremes. Always. Go for either the vamp red or a light, light pink. Maybe black satin if you feel like being goth or punk rock. But do not dip into a middle-ground palette. Corals and fuchsias are just asking for trouble. If you can't decide, go for a clear nail. It will make you look put together and finish off your look in a refined way.

- THE RED: Chanel Vamp (called Rouge Noir in Europe). This shade has never failed me.
- THE LIGHT, LIGHT PINK: Essie Ballet Slippers. Light, easy, feminine, classic.
- THE BLACK: Chanel Black Satin. Hardcore. In a good way.
- THE CLEAR: OPI Designer Series Topcoat. Shows you're ready to take on anything. No fuss, no muss.

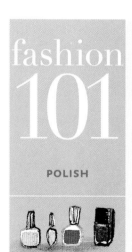

fashion
101

POLISH

Nail polish was invented 5,000 years ago by the Ming Dynasty. Chinese royalty wore colored nail polish according to the colors of the current dynasty (gold and silver during the Chou, red and black during the Ming, etc). Egyptians also stained their nails with the reddish brown henna plant and used polish as signifiers of rank. Queen Nefertiti wore a ruby red and Cleopatra wore a rust red (such stylish queens!), but the lower-ranked women were permitted to use only very pale colors. Obviously, polish used today doesn't signify royalty or rank, but is a matter of taste and appropriateness—so select wisely, as people do notice. I know I do.

60.

Old Concert T-Shirt

THERE ARE FEW THINGS cooler than an old, overworn shirt from a concert by the Stones, the Strokes, the Beatles, the Killers, etc. Every girl has definitely owned a shirt from her favorite band (or bands) to wear with jeans or even under a finely tailored suit (mix of high and low fashion is utterly absorbing, visually). How-Zever, under no circumstances should anyone wear a shirt from a band they do not listen to. Very, very uncool. If you are going to wear the Rolling Stones, you'd better know all the words to "Satisfaction." And in order to wear any band's T-shirt with true style, you must have their albums on your iPod.

That's the rule. Follow it, and rock on.

WITH THE BAND

- These shirts are best when bought at an actual concert. The best fashion pieces come with a story. Authenticity is everything.
- eBay is a good second choice (and since the best concert T-shirts are from the '60s and '70s, it is probably the most sound option).

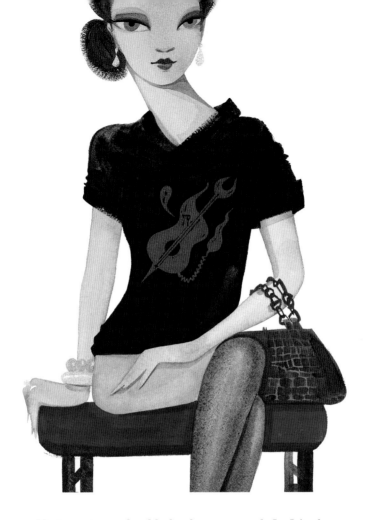

- Vintage stores should also be scavenged. In LA, there are entire stores on Melrose full of vintage T-shirts. In NYC, What Goes Around Comes Around has a good selection. In between, I'm sure your local secondhand store will have a wide selection of T-shirts, and if you're lucky you can find actual originals from time to time. Shop on.

61.

One-Piece Swimsuit

⟨⟨◦⟩⟩

THE BIKINI has become the fashion favorite, but there are some occasions when a bikini is not going to cut it. For these moments a one-piece (or maillot, if we're being proper) is as essential as the little black dress. It can make you appear thinner, cover up areas that may not be bikini-ready or a midsection that has not yet been sun-kissed. It is obviously the way to go if you are vacationing after a Thanksgiving holiday or a New Year's celebration. Hey, even the best of us skip Pilates from time to time.

SUCH OPTIONS!

- Go for an all-black suit. It will always be slimming and elegant. If you can find it with an attachable belt, or pair it up with one of your own choosing, even better.
- An all-white one-piece can be slimming and elegant, too—but just be sure it's not see-through. Beyond tacky.
- Look for suits during the off-season, too. This will take the stress out of having to shop for one that you may need that very afternoon and/or weekend.
- See designers in Bikini (#8) for my favorites!

CLOSET OBSESSION:
ERES SWIMSUITS

Eres swimsuits have been a French institution since 1968, and fashion insiders have been bringing them back from Paris for decades. The appeal of the Eres swimsuit is that the fabric is as light as possible, contours to the body like a second skin, and there is a skill to the cut that magically disguises any flaws. It is impeccably designed to be both flattering and fashionable, and every season the company comes out with a suit that is sure to be the one that the hottest A-list celebrity wears, which then means the piece is completely sold out the very next day. Luckily, you no longer have to be a fashion insider with a plane ticket to Paris to get your hands on one of these suits. In 2000, Eres launched in the United States and has since become a true favorite among American women.

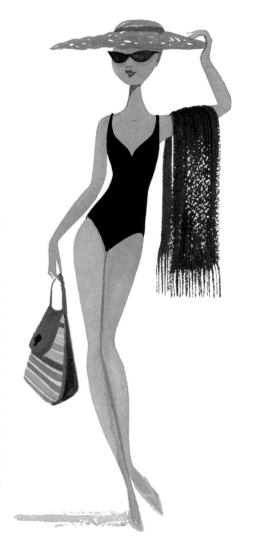

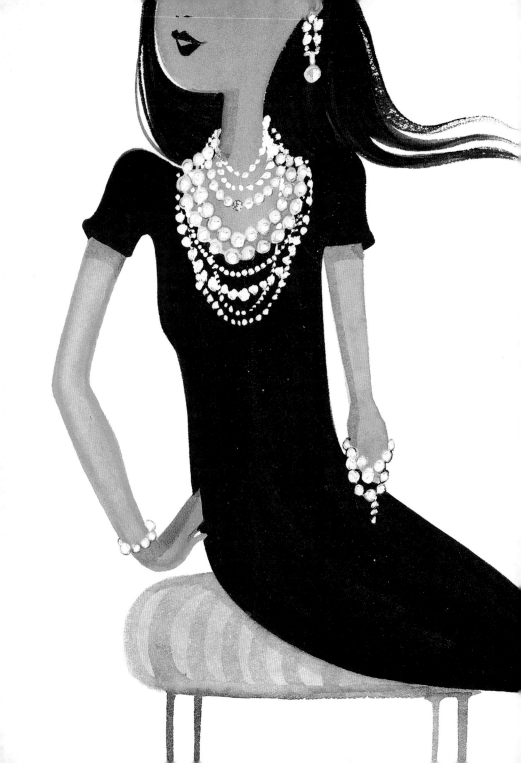

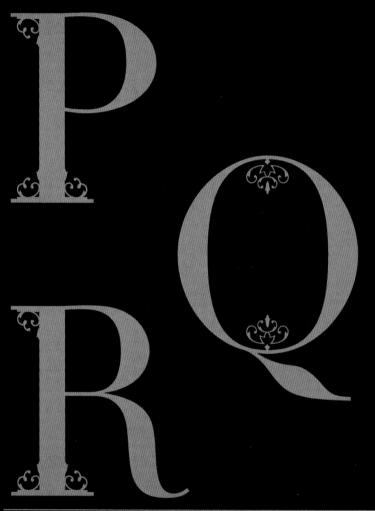

62.
Pajamas

AH, PJs. So restful, so comfortable, *so* must-have. I imagine a pajama-filled world of Greta Garbo and Joan Crawford in wide-legged satin pajamas. I imagine Martha Stewart in blue-and-white monogrammed cotton. Claudette Colbert in oversized versions stolen from her handsome Clark Gable. And Marilyn Monroe in two drops of Chanel N° 5. But the reality is, the world is full of women in sweatpants and flannels and old college T-shirts. This, my friends, should be banned. I know the argument is that the sweatpants and T-shirts are comfortable. But what, I ask, is more comfortable than a pair of pajamas made of silk, satin, or cotton? Nothing.

- SHANGHAI TANG SILK PAJAMAS: A Hong Kong–based luxury-goods company that makes the best traditional Chinese-silk pajamas with the modern twist of adding very bright, unexpected colors.
- FRETTE MEN'S PAJAMAS: Frette is a high-end Italian linen company that moonlights producing splendid his-and-hers pajamas.
- OLATZ SCHNABEL COTTON PAJAMAS: Olatz's bold-colored pajamas made out of sumptuous Egyptian cotton are so magnificent it seems a shame to keep them indoors. But please do. Wearing pajamas out of context is a one-way ticket to fashion disasterdom (unless you are Julian Schnabel!).

Now, just to show you my heart's in the right place,
I'll give you my best pair of pajamas.

CLARK GABLE TO CLAUDETTE COLBERT
IN *IT HAPPENED ONE NIGHT*

63

Peacoat

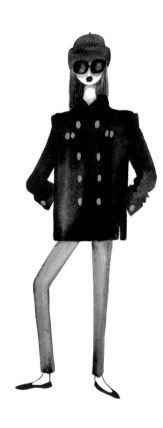

O N COLD WINTER NIGHTS, in the hottest spots in town, there will frequently be a girl walking in wearing a peacoat. She's got that low-key, low-maintenance look about her. When you ask her where she got her coat, she'll probably tell you it's secondhand from the Army-Navy store. Seventy bucks, tops. And you will vow to go in search of your own.

What makes the peacoat so desirable? It's the unfussy practicality about it. Each feature—the warm wool, the double-breasted front, the big buttons (best when anchor-stamped, of course), and those divine oversized lapels—was chosen by the Navy for function, not fashion. The peacoat has been around since the British and Dutch created it 300 years ago, and has lasted through three centuries of naval wear and round-the-globe treks, so it's safe to say it's got some staying power. Most definitely.

WHERE OH WHERE DO I GET ONE?

- The Army-Navy store has the best. Go to the source, if you can.
- If want to look elsewhere, the classic shape has been redone by everyone from H&M to YSL. But keep it as close to the original as possible so that it will last you season after season.
- Make sure the fabric is a stiff wool. You don't want a soft cotton fabric, because then you lose that firm collar, which is the best part of the whole coat (in my opinion).
- Go for the classic colors: navy, black, gray, or loden green. Any other color just looks like it came from an alternate universe.
- The proportions should be a little wide and a little oversized. This is one coat you don't want to be too tailored.

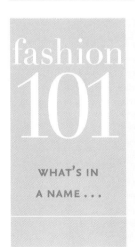

fashion
101

WHAT'S IN
A NAME . . .

The term "peacoat" comes from the Dutch word *pij*, which is a type of cloth often used in making the coat.

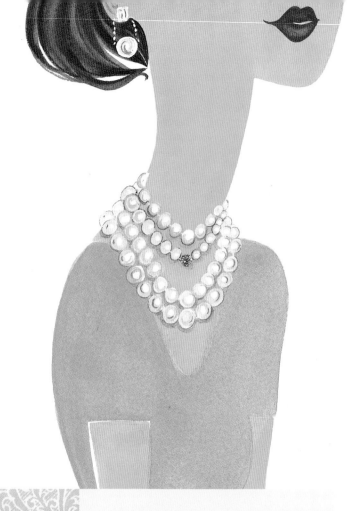

FUN FACTS

- **1916:** Jeweler Jacques Cartier bought his Manhattan store by trading a double strand of cultured pearls for the building.
- **1996:** Jackie O's $80 strand of fake pearls sold at auction for $211,500.

64.
Pearl Necklace

PEARLS ARE WONDERFUL when layered in long, opera-length strands. (Google *Coco Chanel in her pearls*. Or the 2005 Lanvin show. Or 1920s socialite Sara Murphy, who wore her pearls to the beach every day—shouldn't we all!) But if you wear pearls in a precious way or take them too seriously, they lose their cool. You have to get creative and don't let 'em get too snooty. Wear them with a paper-thin tank top and a dangerously high heel. Or mix them in with your junk jewelry or thick biker chains. They can be real or they can be fake. It really doesn't matter—but they must never, ever be haughty.

WHERE TO BUY

- MIKIMOTO. If you have the money, this is the best.
- LANVIN ON GROSGRAIN RIBBON. These necklaces are so amazing that they single-handedly put Lanvin back in the fashion spotlight in 2005.
- EBAY or your local costume jewelry store, for cheap fabulous fakes.
- MY FAVORITES ARE baroque (irregularly shaped) pearls that are imperfect and come in colors besides white.

65.
Pencil Skirt

A PENCIL SKIRT immediately conjures up images of femmes fatales—the best film noir has to offer. There is a power about the pencil skirt, a certain sophistication. But there is also a subversive sexuality as it manages to show off the legs without showing them at all. What an illusion! It asserts femininity, but it also asserts power, which is the best feature a skirt can have: powerful femininity. And the savvy, stylish woman is well aware of this combination. She takes deliberate steps, strides confidently by in her high heels, and pretends to be oblivious to the stir her pencil skirt is causing.

While clothes may not make the woman, they certainly have a strong effect on her self-confidence—which, I believe, does make the woman.

MARY KAY ASH

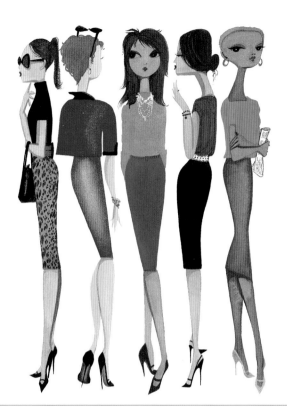

PENCILING IT IN

- The hemline should fall just below or just above the knee.
- It is most flattering when worn with sky-high heels.
- Try a high-waisted version to elongate the line of the body.
- It should always be snug but never *too* tight.
- It should have a vent or it could be hard to walk or sit. Be mindful of such tailoring.
- A little stretch in the fabric makes it immeasurably easier to wear.

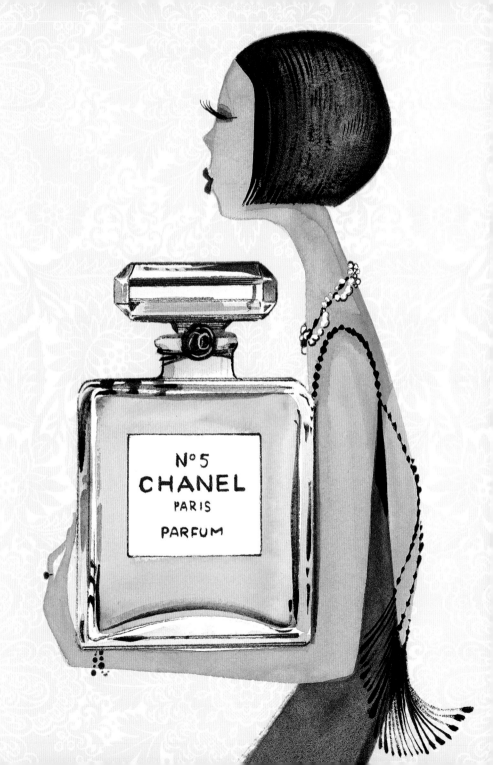

66.
Perfume

PERFUME is a powerful weapon. It can take you back in an instant, transporting you to moments in time—long-ago summers, the beach, first kisses, old lovers.

Some women have a perfume for day and a perfume for night; others change it by the season. Some try a new fragrance every time a celebrity attaches her name to one; others have been wearing the same scent since they were sixteen.

Personally, I think it is best to find a signature scent and stick to it, so when that old lover steps into the elevator and smells your scent, he'll remember the one that got away. . .

A woman who does not wear perfume has no future.

COCO CHANEL

THESE ARE A FEW TIME-TESTED FAVORITES:

- Santa Maria Novella colognes: Santa Maria Novella is one of the world's oldest and most beloved apothecaries. They are based out of Florence and have been since 1221. Their Acqua di Colonia is perhaps the favorite among their scents and is known as "The Queen's Cologne," as it was reputedly created for Catherine de Medici.
- Fracas: A sweet floral fragrance, created by Robert Piguet in 1948. It has been a cult smash among women in the know for decades (e.g., Madonna, Martha Stewart, Sofia Coppola).
- Any man's cologne: Many of the world's most fashionable and intriguing women famously wear men's cologne (e.g., Angelina Jolie, Elle Macpherson, and Carine Roitfeld).
- Chanel N° 5: But of course.

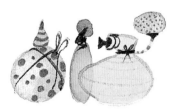

FUN FACT
One bottle of Chanel N° 5 is sold every thirty seconds.

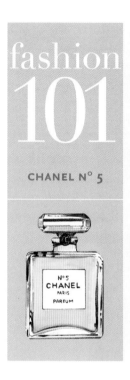

fashion 101

CHANEL N° 5

In 1920, Coco Chanel decided, "I want to give women an artificial perfume. Yes, I really do mean artificial, like a dress, something that has been made. I don't want any rose or lily of the valley, I want a perfume that is a composition." That year, she commissioned Ernest Beaux to create six "artificial" scents. After testing all six, Chanel decided that N° 5 was her favorite and thus, the famous formula was born. It was the first perfume to use large amounts of synthetic substances and aldehydes. Before use of synthetics, perfume would have to be applied very heavily or frequently reapplied throughout the evening. But Chanel N° 5 stuck with a woman all night, and in turn, women have stuck with Chanel N° 5 for almost a century. It's the perfect codependent relationship.

Where should one wear perfume?
Wherever one wants to be kissed.

COCO CHANEL

67.
Plain White Tee

⟿⟾

I AM OBSESSED WITH Hanes three-packs. They cost nothing and will last a long time. But a sea change occurred with our plain white tees: It has recently gone the way of our plain blue jeans. There is a new T-shirt designer every other week. And everyone struggles to keep up with who "the" T-shirt is, or "Where is it made? Peru or China?" or "How aged does it look?" These days it has to be *barely there*—the thinner and lighter the better. It has to look old and vintage, though the brand ironically changes week by week. I like a great thin white T-shirt as much as the next girl. And yes, I occasionally will buy "the" brand of the week. But I refuse to obsess over something that is supposed to indicate a cool, casual ease. So for the most part, I'm sticking with my Hanes. Simple is sometimes the best route to take on this one.

THE INSIDE TRACK: **MY FAVORITES**

- Hanes: The old staple . . . inexpensive and perfectly basic.
- James Perse: Perse may be responsible for starting the luxury T-shirt craze. The high-quality/low-maintenance look is the hallmark of the brand.
- Adam + Eve: Available in an array of colors. I love the ones that look washed out, as if they'd been sitting in the sun.

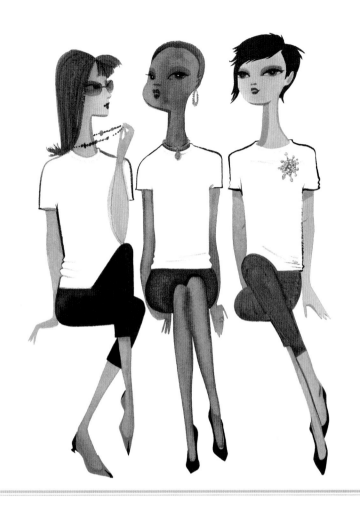

I've always thought of the T-shirt as
the alpha and the omega of the fashion alphabet.

GIORGIO ARMANI

- The Row: Light and thin—almost too thin—tees that demand to be layered. The brand also plays with proportions and lengths, also a great layering feature.
- Rick Owens: Nobody does casual cool like Rick Owens. His T-shirts are clingy, superfine, and worth every penny. They epitomize his self-titled "glunge" (glamour plus grunge) look.
- Vince: Their butter-soft T-shirts—just one of the luxe basics the company makes—have become an iconic American original since they debuted in 2003.
- C&C California: A T-shirt brand that truly embodies California chic: laid-back, comfy, cool, and not afraid of a bit of color.

IT'S NOT JUST A T-SHIRT!

- Pay attention to the neckline. It should not come up too high or go down too low.
- Never wear a too-tight T-shirt. It should hang a little loose on the body.
- Use it to dress down a suit (or to dress down almost anything, for that matter).
- Bottom line: You want it to look like you just threw it on and didn't think about it. Effortlessness must be a part of any stylish woman's arsenal.

68.
Polo Shirt

⌘

THE POLO SHIRT, true to its name, was designed to be worn on the polo field. It became standard issue at the country club and became a part of the prepster/geek uniform: khakis, oxfords, and polos (collar up!). It found its way into the urban jungle when the fashionistas began embracing all things prep and geek. Of course, to give it a fashion look, the prepster/geek uniform should not be copied too literally; it should be stepped up into an entirely new fashion level. (Note: No uniform should ever be copied too literally—everything has to be stepped up and made unique. *Everything*.) So instead of wearing a polo with khakis and oxfords, pair it with jeans tucked into riding boots and an of-the-moment jacket. Or wear it a size too small (think Scarlett Johansson in *Lost in Translation*). Or, when you do wear it with khakis, make sure they are big and rumpled (see Khakis, #44). When you wear a polo shirt as a style item, you must follow the cardinal rule of fashion: something always has to be off, slightly amiss, askew. Imperfection is the perfect road to honing your signature look and point of view.

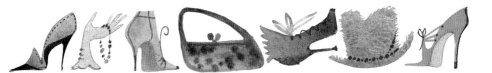

PREPPY LE PEW

- Try it in both classic colors (white, navy) and bright colors (orange, royal blue).
- Try layering one on top of the other. On the right person, this can be very chic.
- Consider going down a size. You want it to hug your body, not drape.
- Consider the long-sleeved versions too. They are often overlooked, but in my opinion, they are even more stylish.

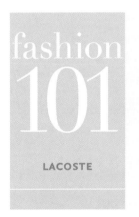

fashion
101

LACOSTE

The polo shirt was strictly athletic wear until René Lacoste, an international tennis champion, asked a friend to design a short-sleeve cotton-knit shirt to wear on the court. Before the Lacoste shirt was made, tennis was played in uncomfortable long-sleeved woven shirts. Lacoste's nickname was "*le crocodile*," and so the little croc was placed on the left breast as the logo. This is reportedly the first instance of a brand logo being sewn on the outside of a piece of clothing. We've not been without that adorable crocodile ever since.

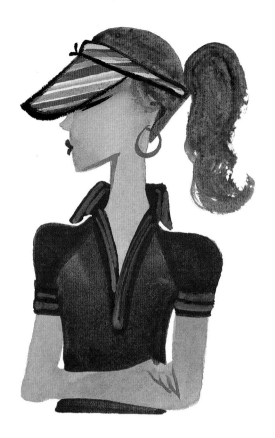

POLOS AND THEIR LOGOS

- Lacoste: The original polo, with the notorious crocodile logo (est. 1933).
- Fred Perry: A laurel logo sewn on the left breast (est. 1952).
- Ralph Lauren: The ever-recognizable polo player logo (est. 1972).
- Rugby Ralph Lauren: A small skull where the polo player usually rides (est. 2004).

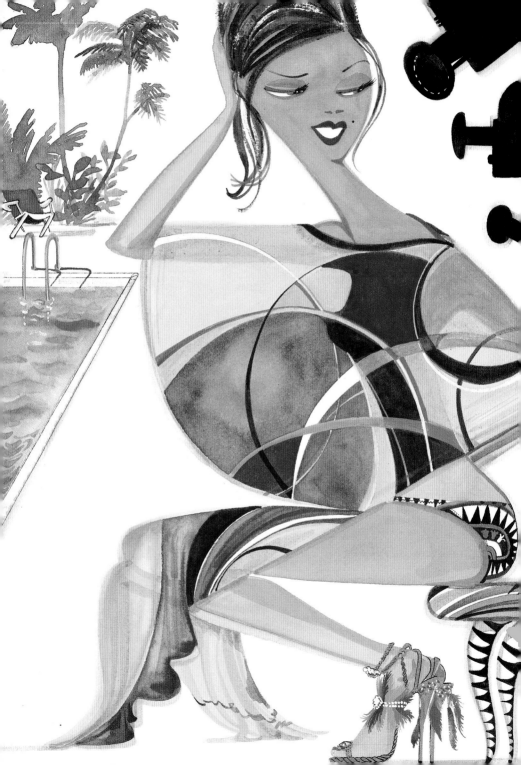

69.
Pucci

A PUCCI PRINT conjures up images of the enviable jet-setters of the '60s. As they stepped onto their private planes, they always seemed to be photographed in bright, bold Pucci dresses. They were the women who refused to fade into the background, who refused to be plain Janes, who knew that style was about standing out a bit. And though those days of '60s jet-setters are long gone, Pucci prints remain—stronger, bolder than ever.

Today, wearing the designer is just as chic and just as enviable as it was back then. Even a small piece of Pucci—a scarf in your hair or tied to your bag—will make you look just a little bit '60s jet-set. But if you want to go full throttle, go for the dress. It will always be the secret missile in your summer arsenal. You don't have to wear it every summer. Put it on ice for a year or two. But then, when you bring it out and unleash it, the dress is going to make the same impression it did when you first put it on. *Blast off.* And best of all, it's still going to look so *right now*. Pucci always does.

Elegance is good taste plus a dash of daring.

CARMEL SNOW

THE PERFECT PUCCI

- A Pucci scarf is a good way to display a piece of the designer for a smaller price tag.
- If you wear a Pucci dress, make sure your accessories do not compete.
- The original Pucci dresses were hand-signed. If you ever see one in a vintage store, snag it. It's almost priceless.

fashion
101

EMILIO PUCCI:

THE PRINCE

OF PRINTS

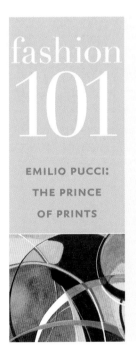

Emilio Pucci was on the slopes in St. Moritz when a *Harper's Bazaar* photographer asked to photograph him in his self-designed ski pants. Pucci, a former Olympic skier, then burst onto the fashion scene quite by accident. This burst came in the 1950s, when styles were constrictive and structured. Pucci broke the mold and started creating jersey-silk dresses that were decidedly unstructured. He became known for the bright colors and bold prints used to make his garments. His dresses became a high-society staple, loved for the daring style and perhaps because they were a perfect travel garment (weighing in at a mere three to four ounces and wonderfully wrinkle-free). The globe-trotting gal was never without one.

70.

Push-Up Bra

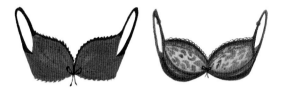

NAMED ONE OF the greatest inventions of the twentieth century, the push-up bra is a universally adored item, which bestows cleavage where there once was none. A girl must choose wisely when and where she wears such a bra. A first date, probably. A job interview, probably not. And in general, no matter where you go, the cleavage should be mostly concealed. Less is more . . . unless you are trying to get out of a speeding ticket.

CLOSET OBSESSION: **PUSH KIN**

- La Perla: This luxury company makes lavish bras that are worth the investment.
- Kiki de Montparnasse: Pushes the envelope on sexuality.
- Agent Provocateur: Pushes the envelope even further.
- Victoria's Secret: An affordable option. They come in a variety of styles and colors.
- Wonderbra: The one that started it all. See Fashion 101.

fashion
101

LADIES AND GENTLEMEN, THE WONDERBRA

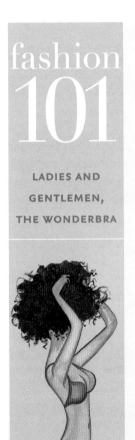

In 1994, a British-born bra descended on the United States with a mania usually reserved for British-born bands. The first Wonderbras arrived in Manhattan in armored cars and limousines. Models, bodyguards, and security guards unloaded the boxes as throngs of women tossed confetti and waved signs. In Miami, the bras rolled in by pink Cadillac. In San Francisco, they arrived by cable car. And in LA, by helicopter.

They sold at a rate of one every fifteen seconds and produced a cultural phenomenon like no other. They also produced some pretty amazing journalistic quotes and marketing slogans:

BEST HEADLINE

We can talk about this calmly.

LOS ANGELES TIMES

BEST WONDERBRA SLOGAN

Look me in the eyes
and tell me that you love me.

BEST CELEBRITY ENDORSEMENT

I swear, even I get cleavage with them.

KATE MOSS

71.
Quality Champagne

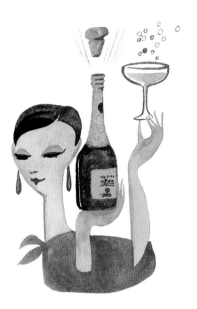

MARK TWAIN ONCE SAID, "Too much of anything is bad, but too much Champagne is just right." Maybe he didn't mean it as a style tip, but we can certainly take it as one, can't we? Champagne is the drink of celebration, and therefore, one should always have a bottle ready and waiting. It should be opened for big occasions, small occasions, or no occasion at all. Life is too short to save our best clothes or our best Champagne for the big events. Drink up. No one can say no to bubbles.

- MOËT HENNESSY: The company dates back to 1743 and was the Champagne of Napoleon and Jefferson and Queen Elizabeth. In 1987, it fashionably merged with Louis Vuitton. What a pair indeed!
- MOËT ET CHANDON'S DOM PERIGNON: Named after the monk Dom Perignon, who is often erroneously credited with discovering Champagne. The story goes that he said, "Come quickly. I am dancing the stars." Apparently the story is false. However, it is a good quote (and a great Champagne).

There comes a time in every woman's life when the only thing that helps is a glass of Champagne.

BETTE DAVIS

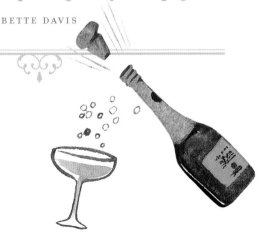

72.
Red Lipstick

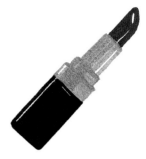

OTHING SAYS Hollywood glamour like a red lip. Every actress, model, and style icon lays claim to a tube or two. And all these women will tell you they know the best red lipstick. They've spent hours at the cosmetics counter and have it figured out. It's Chanel Red No. 5. Or MAC Ruby Woo. Or Clinique Angel Red. Cover Girl Really Red. Lancôme Red Desire. Anna Sui Rouge Chine. Mary Kay Red Salsa. Elizabeth Arden Slink. NARS Fire Down Below. Trucco Blood Red. Etc., etc.

Yes, clearly everyone has it figured out.

The fact of the matter is you have to spend an afternoon hitting the cosmetics counter yourself. Red lipstick is much like the little black dress or your favorite pair of jeans. One size does *not* fit all. Skin tones and lip size and face shape all play a role. So, you just have to try them all on and then take a good, long look at yourself in the mirror. Much like the perfect dress or the perfect pair of jeans, you will know when you've found "the one." And then you, too, can tell everyone that you have this red lipstick thing all figured out. You know the very best one. In my case, it's Chanel Red No. 5.

If you don't wear lipstick, I can't talk to you.

THE LATE, GREAT ISABELLA BLOW

HOW TO *WEAR* RED LIPSTICK

- Choose the right shade of red. For fair skin, go for a red that has blue undertones. For ruddy skin, choose a pinkish red. Olive skin looks best with warm reds that have an orange, gold, or brown base. Dark brown skin is stunning in a bright fuchsia-red. But of course, confer with the women at the cosmetics counter.
- Keep the rest of the makeup simple. Red lipstick is statement enough. Don't overdo the eye makeup or the blush or you run the risk of looking like a clown. Let the lips be the focus.
- Make sure you know how to apply it. It is a bit of an art form. This is not the lipstick you can throw on in the back of a taxi. Again, confer with the women at the cosmetics counter and also see below.

Beauty, to me, is about being comfortable in your own skin. That, or a kick-ass red lipstick.

GWYNETH PALTROW

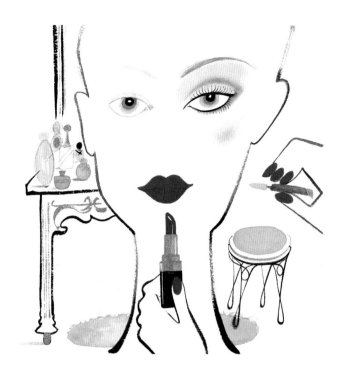

HOW TO *APPLY* RED LIPSTICK

- Apply a lip moisturizer first and then a thin layer of foundation.
- After the foundation dries, add a layer of face powder, which will help set the lipstick so that it will last longer.
- Next, line the lips with a pencil that matches your lip-stick. Keep within the natural line of your lip.
- Apply a thin, even coat of the lipstick.
- Blot. Always remember to blot!
- Apply a second coat and you're ready to go.

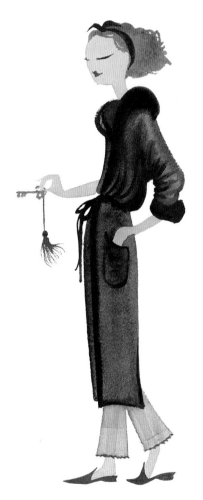

73.
Robe

⟨⟨∞⟩⟩

A SILK ROBE is an essential garment for after-baths or morning-afters. If one accidentally gets locked out of her apartment, one should always be wearing only the best robe. I always admire a woman who looks good in her loungewear. She is the woman who can lose the key to her hotel room and glamorously walk to the lobby without giving it a second thought. (Note: She usually has the good pajamas to go underneath and the good slippers to match.) There is no shame or embarrassment. She can even stop at the lobby bar, if she so desires. I'd like to think we can all be this woman. And really, all it takes is a good silk robe (and the pajamas and slippers). Is that really so difficult?

ROBE IT!

- Cotton, cashmere, and silk are the three standards. No terry cloth, no no *no* chenille!
- When choosing a silk robe, keep it simple. No flowers, no lace, no designs. Or you'll look like a mental patient.
- Wearing a man's silk robe is a really sexy option. Makes people wonder what you were doing just a few minutes ago.
- Consider a vintage silk kimono from Chinatown for a unique option. Here, flowers are OK!
- Don't you dare wear a terry cloth robe that is five times too big. It's going to make you look twenty pounds heavier. Bad, bad, bad.
- Where to buy? See Pajamas (#62).

Give me my robe, put on my crown;
I have immortal longings in me.

CLEOPATRA,
FROM SHAKESPEARE'S *ANTONY AND CLEOPATRA*

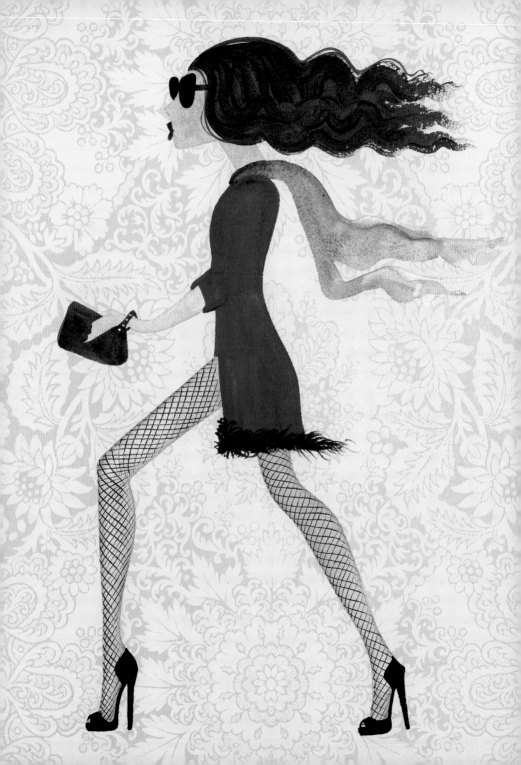

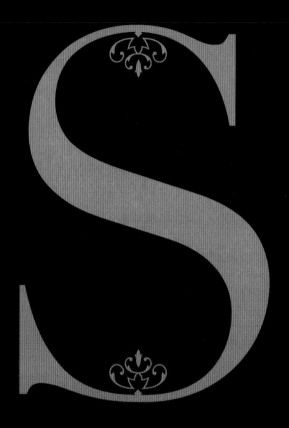

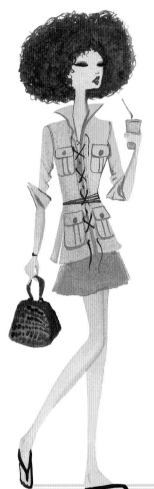

74.

Safari Jacket

⟨⟩⟨⟩⟨⟩

THE SAFARI JACKET still conjures up images of wealthy people going on safari in Africa, which is perhaps why it has maintained its appeal for over fifty years. I love the look. So very Veruschka in YSL. Who doesn't want to look like she is going on safari in Kenya, even if she is just running out to Starbucks? A safari jacket is one of those items that has always been a regular in the runway rotation. Maybe it will skip a season or two, but it always comes back.

We must never confuse elegance with snobbery.

YVES SAINT LAURENT

BIG-GAME HUNTER

- Don't take it too literally. Don't go to Abercrombie & Kent for the authentic one. Instead look for versions that have been altered for fashion appeal: cropped styles, short sleeves, tucks and pleats.
- If you want to sound like a fashion snob, call it a *Saharienne*, which is the name taken from YSL's original collection.
- You can almost always find a good version at Michael Kors or Banana Republic.
- As always with something that is decidedly masculine, pair it with something decidedly feminine for a fashionable contrast.
- Also a great alternative to the Blazer (#11).

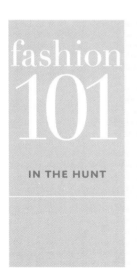

fashion
101

IN THE HUNT

It was meant to be a jacket for going on safaris and probably dates back to the 1800s, when British military officials wore it in tropical climates. In the '60s, the once-utilitarian jacket began to trek down runways and into the urban jungle. It was in the hands of Yves Saint Laurent (the master!) that the piece turned into a fashion monument. In 1968, the designer debuted his Saharienne collection, and he revealed the first high-fashion safari jacket. That same year, fashion model Veruschka's boyfriend photographed her wearing the YSL jacket with a miniskirt, a tattered hat, and a hip-slung belt. It was the shot seen round the world, and the safari jacket became a must-have item ever since.

75.

Sandals

⸺∞∞∞⸺

I THINK IT IS MANDATORY that every woman have two pairs of summertime sandals: a casual daytime pair and a dressy nighttime pair. For the day, a gladiator sandal will always be chic and stylish (though some seasons it gets more attention than others). The low version of the gladiator sandal is classic and enduring. The up-to-the-knee version (Google *Mary-Kate Olsen in gladiators*) has its days in the sun and then fades away for a few years. For night, a metallic sandal will match every single summertime outfit. For low-key summer nights, a flat metallic thong is perfection. But when you are kicking it up a notch, the heels should come up with you. A metallic stiletto sandal (gold or silver) is really the only option for a summer night on the town.

FOOT FETISH

- Your sandals must fit as perfectly as your best stilettos. No part of the foot should spill over the side or front or back.
- Make sure your feet are perfectly pedicured. *Please!* Remember this, if nothing else.

K. JACQUES

The K. Jacques company was created in 1933 by Mr. and Mrs. Keklikian Jacques. Their sandals represent authentic Saint-Tropez fashion. They are cool and casual and radiate the relaxed, tranquil Mediterranean atmosphere. It is still a family business today, all of the products are made in France, and the brand has three stores in Saint-Tropez and a boutique in the Le Marais quarter of Paris. However, the sandals can also be found at high-end department stores and online. They were a hit early on with celebrities and the fashion elite. They continue to be favorites today and will endure as long as cool and casual Saint-Tropez styles are in vogue (i.e., until the end of time).

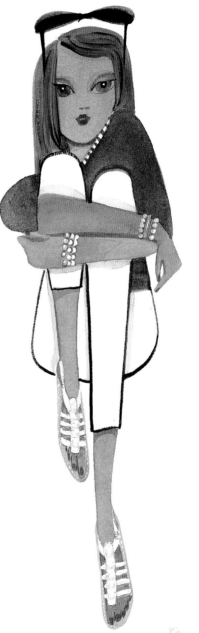

CLOSET OBSESSION: **JACK ROGERS**

Jack Rogers Navajo sandals are a beloved beach and resort staple. The moccasin-inspired design of the thong sandal was the invention of a Florida cobbler who made them for an upscale store in Palm Beach. Jack Rogers Navajos were at first a local hit and now are a worldwide obsession. They are made in every color and material imaginable (crocodile, suede, alligator, python), and the signature whip-stitching makes for plenty of color combos. You can get them custom-made, monogrammed, high-heeled or low-heeled, and they are a must for channeling Jackie O, Kate Hudson, or Liv Tyler in all their summer glory.

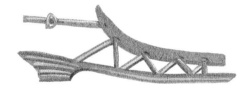

Direct your feet to the sunny side of the street . . .

DOROTHY FIELDS

76.

Sarong

WRAPPING A BEACH TOWEL around you is not nearly as fashionable (or flattering) as wrapping yourself in a silk sarong. The cotton versions are great, too. A sarong is an essential poolside or beachside accessory. It can be wrapped around the neck or knotted on one hip or be worn as a turban or do double-duty as a towel. It can become a dress, a shawl, or even a bag. Women who are well practiced in the art of tying the sarong are capable of changing it from a daytime cover-up to a casual evening dress to wear to dinner or to drinks. Women who are not experts should perhaps secure the sarong with a brooch . . . you can never be too sure. One thing is certain, though: Its options are endless.

WHERE TO BUY . . .

- The sarong is a traditional garment worn by men and women in Malaysia and India, so good ethnic shops will have plenty to choose from.
- If you must go high-end, Hermès and Eres are good options.

- Calypso makes good versions and always has some in stock.
- Any vacation town will have them in its boutiques.
- Whether it is Hermès or Eres, it is more about "what corner of the world it is from."

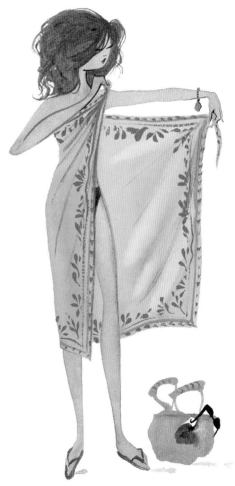

77.

Signet Ring

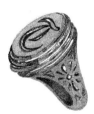

IN THE ANCIENT WORLD, the signet ring was like your credit card or BlackBerry—if you lost it, you'd go into a state of panic. Back then, your signet ring functioned as your signature and was used to seal contracts. Today, it has a power all its own. It is an indicator of your individuality, because each ring is engraved exactly as you want it to be. The classic version has your family crest, school insignia, or monogram (usually all three initials). But if you feel like being less traditional, you can have anything from an inside joke to a milestone inscribed. Perhaps the initials of your alter ego?

SIGNED, SEALED, DELIVERED . . .

- If you don't mind wearing someone else's initials or family crest, search antique jewelry stores, where you will find old, intricately designed signets.
- Tiffany has great signet rings, if you want to go classic.
- Like a cocktail ring, it can go on any finger you choose.

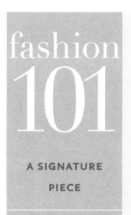

fashion
101

A SIGNATURE
PIECE

Traditionally, the signet ring was one's signature, and stealing a signet ring was a serious offense. The mark on the ring could either enhance one's reputation or condemn one to death (e.g., if you wore a ring with the impression of Brutus and Cassius after Julius Caesar's assassination).

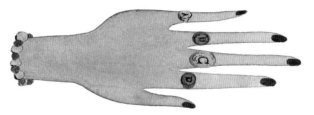

FUN FACTS

- Women of rank in the Middle Ages wore signet rings as symbols of prestige.
- Michelangelo's famous signet ring had a carving of a segment of the Sistine Chapel.
- Dreaming of a signet ring boded well or ill, depending on the nature of the dream. Either way, dreaming about one is a sure sign that change is a-brewing.

78.

Silk Scarf

THE ONLY WAY to really understand the value of a scarf is to spend an afternoon at a Parisian café and just watch the women walk by. Scarves as belts, scarves decorating handbags, scarves as tops, scarves as headbands, scarves tied through the back loops of trench coats, scarves tied around the neck in eighty-eight different ways, and on and on and on. It does seem, as is so often said, that the women of Paris are born knowing how to wear a scarf. The rest of us have to watch and learn and maybe seek out an instructional guide or two. In 1988, Jean-Louis Dumas-Hermès put out a pictorial pamphlet called "How to Wear Your Hermès Scarf." If you can manage to find it, it is the most inspiring manual. But if you cannot get your hands on the pamphlet or a plane ticket to Paris, you're just going to have to resort to good old-fashioned practice.

FUN FACT

An Hermès scarf is sold somewhere in the world every twenty-five seconds.

ALL TIED UP

- In addition to Hermès, Gucci and Ferragamo make beautiful printed silk scarves. These are traditional, iconic souvenirs from one's first trip to Italy. They are instant heirlooms.
- Consider it as a piece of jewelry and wear it as such (it should add oomph and drama).
- It should be personal and a part of you—it doesn't have to be silk if that's not your thing.

NOTABLE APPEARANCES

- As Grace Kelly's sling to support her broken arm
- As Queen Elizabeth's neckwear in a 1950s postage stamp
- As Jackie O's publicity shield throughout the '60s
- As Audrey Hepburn's hat decoration in *Breakfast at Tiffany's*
- As Sharon Stone's shackles in *Basic Instinct*
- As Madonna's halter in *Swept Away*
- As Sarah Jessica Parker's bandana in *Sex and the City*

CLOSET OBSESSION: **THE HERMÈS SCARF**

It is just 90 centimeters and 65 grams of silk, yet it takes two years to create a single Hermès scarf. Technically, the process begins in Brazil, where the silk is spun from cocoons woven by the larvae of 250 silk moths. As the silk is spinning in Brazil, the design process begins in Lyon, France, where all of the designers are briefed on what the theme of the season's collection will be. Then, over fifty artists create designs for the ten scarves to be produced that season. After the many months it takes to create the designs, an engraver will make a silk screen for each different color that will appear on each scarf. If there are thirty colors in one scarf, he must create thirty different silk screens. Then there is an intensive coloration process, as an entire committee will vote on the shades and tones, before the design is finally sent to the factory where the dirty work begins. There is a dizzying printing process, then a luxurious steam bath to make the scarves unbelievably soft, and then two women painstakingly scrutinize each centimeter of silk for any defects. Last, the squares are cut and seamstresses edge them by hand, before they are shipped off to be snatched up by women the world over.

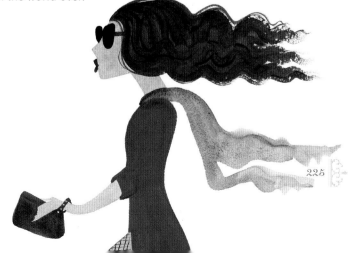

79.

Slippers

A FTER SPENDING HOURS in high heels, your feet deserve to be pampered in something cloudlike. Puffy and comfy, a slipper should be as comfortable as possible, and luxury is recommended. Find a pair lined in sheepskin or fleece for the winter. Or go very high-end and get a mink pair (which also makes a great gift, by the way). Or you can get a super-silly marabou pair for being sexy at home. Or go Moroccan-style, which lets you run out to the grocery store without looking like a nut. I guess you could hop down that so popular bunny-slippered road, which is not the sexiest road in the world, and which will *definitely* make you look like a nut at the grocery store. But who am I to judge? *wink*

*It's easier to put on slippers
than to carpet the whole world.*

AL FRANKEN

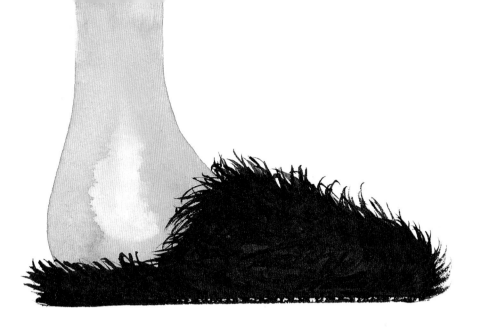

CLOSET OBSESSION: **STUBBS & WOOTTON**

Stubbs & Woottons are the most divine handmade slippers. They are not just comfortable; they also have innovative and inventive needlepoint designs on the front (e.g., skull and crossbones, Maryland crabs, polo players being thrown from their horses), which earn plenty of compliments when worn around the house or on the street. Yes, you can wear these outdoors. They are made of the finest fabrics: English leather, Egyptian cotton, French brocade, and Belgian needlepoint. They are comfy, which is a necessary quality for slippers. But S&Ws will also garner you genuine compliments when you run to the store for a pint of ice cream.

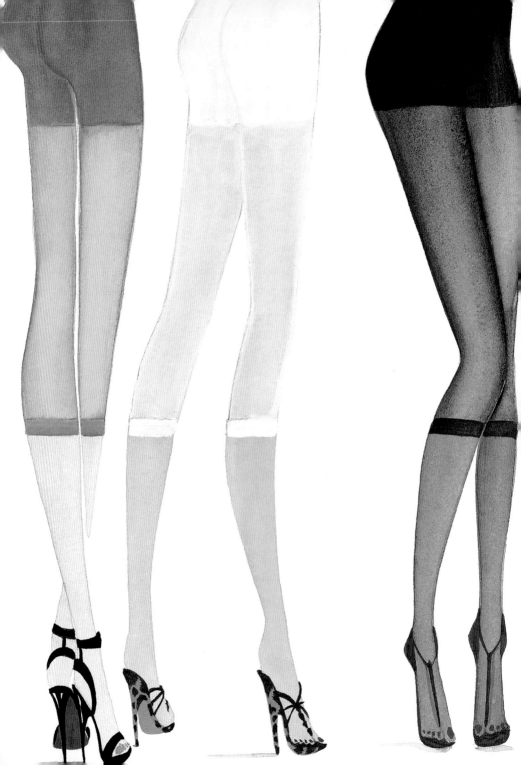

80.

Spanx

A LIFE-ALTERING, footless, control-top panty hose that should be worn whenever a woman wants to appear a size smaller. Celebrities raved about them from the moment they hit the market. Oprah featured them on her show as one of her "favorite things." Gwyneth Paltrow told a reporter her secret for looking red-carpet ready: "There are these great things called Spanx . . . they just squeeze you in. It's terrific. All the Hollywood girls do it." The Spanx secret spread quickly, and if they are not in every woman's drawer, they damn well should be.

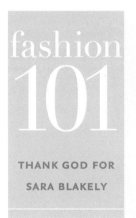

fashion
101

THANK GOD FOR
SARA BLAKELY

Seven years ago Sara Blakely was selling copiers and fax machines door-to-door. Today, she is every woman's favorite inventor. Her idea for Spanx was born out of a bit of frustration and a bit of innovation. One night, on an impulse, she cut the feet out of her pantyhose to wear under white pants. She discovered that she looked slimmer, everything was smoothed out, there was no panty line. So she cleared her bank account of $5,000 and set out to change the world. Mission accomplished.

81.
Statement Necklace

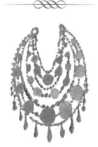

A STATEMENT NECKLACE is large and bold (some can even be incredibly theatrical and dramatic—in a good way). The statement necklace is the fashion equivalent of a supporting actress that steals the show. When done well, this can be a beautiful thing to see. The top echelon of Hollywood starlets will all agree that sometimes it is best to let the accessory take center stage (think Jennifer Garner, Nicole Kidman, and Cate Blanchett at the 2008 Oscars). But on the red carpet, statement necklaces cost a pretty penny (which is why they are usually borrowed) and make a more serious statement. On the street, they can be inexpensive and speak a totally different language.

As with the cocktail ring, the necklace should be big, and need not be real. And it's best if you own several. The beauty of owning a collection of statement jewelry (real or fake) is that they let you wear your standby Little Black Dress (#48) time after time, pushing your look further and further into that of the desired fashionista. Your look will never get tired when coupled with the right statement necklace. Ever.

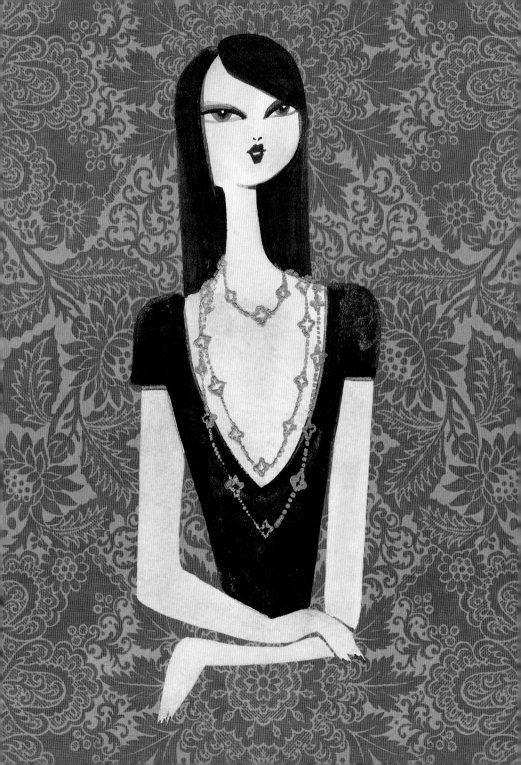

STATE YOUR CASE

- Hold off on the statement necklace when you're wearing your Pucci (#69). It's best with a plain backdrop. Sometimes, too much is simply too much. Always remember this.
- This is a must when traveling—you can pack two dresses and three statement necklaces, and get by for a week.
- A good statement necklace is your ultimate "quick-change" item. If you need an outfit to go from conservative to avant-garde in sixty seconds flat, a statement necklace and a good pair of stilettos (#82) are all you need.

THE INSIDE TRACK: **MY FAVORITES**

The statement necklace talks. It tells the world a little bit about a girl. It establishes a vibe and paints a picture. A few that are mainstays on the magazine pages include:

- Tom Binns: For the pop princess spreads.
- Van Cleef & Arpels: For the ultimate uptown spreads.
- Marni: For the fashionable boho spreads.
- Oversized beads or ethnic designs from the Moroccan flea market: For the original boho spreads.

82.

Stilettos

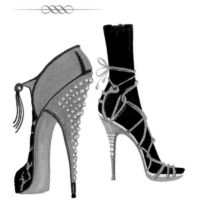

THIS SHOE IS CAPABLE OF invoking euphoria, admiration, panic, and justifiable credit card debt. You can never have too many stilettos, and you'll never feel as though you have enough. Ask the notorious Imelda Marcos. In 1986, when she fled the Philippines with her dictator husband, news reports came through that she left behind three thousand pairs of shoes in her closet. (She later said she left behind only one thousand and sixty, but who's counting?) Much of the world balked—but I've gotta say, I wanted to meet the woman, as I think she lived out a shoe fantasy most women would kill for. More accurately, I wanted to see her stiletto collection. A woman's entire being can be understood by the heels she turns on.

What's more is that the stiletto helps to define the curvature of a woman's leg, and offers height, confidence, and sass. A woman wearing the right stiletto is a true force to be reckoned with.

INVEST, INVEST, INVEST

The names you hear time and again—Manolo Blahnik, Jimmy Choo, Christian Louboutin—you hear for a reason. They know what they are doing. They know how to create a classic, timeless shoe and make four-inch heels that are actually comfortable to walk in. Geniuses, all of them. But genius does not come cheap. I know some people think it is ridiculous to spend so much money on a pair of shoes. I'll tell you why it is not:

- Quality, expensive shoes will last longer and wear better.
- They will not leave you hobbling down the street.
- You will feel incredible every time you slip them on.

HOW TO WALK IN STILETTOS

1. Practice.
2. Practice.
3. Practice.

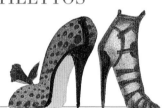

How many pairs of shoes do you need?

MEN

83.
Striped Sailor Shirt

N o self-respecting Frenchwoman, Frenchman, or French film lacks a striped sailor shirt. Jean Paul Gaultier seems to always be wearing one. And one of Gaultier's models will usually parade down the catwalk in some sort of version of the shirt, every time. The images of Jean Seberg wearing hers in the classic 1960s film *Breathless* (a must-watch) will never be forgotten. Picasso gave it artistic cachet, Bardot wore one as a cover-up—the list of Frenchmen and French-women in this shirt is endless. The striped sailor shirt is one of those items that embodies French chic, and it completely disarms that old myth that horizontal stripes are not flattering. When they are worn with a boatneck and French attitude, they are the most flattering lines in the world.

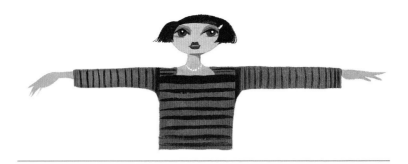

SAIL AWAY

YOU WILL ALWAYS BE ABLE TO FIND A STRIPED SAILOR SHIRT AT THESE SHOPS:

- PETIT BATEAU: For the classic version.
- L.L.BEAN: For the old standby.
- JEAN PAUL GAULTIER: For the designer option.
- ARMOR LUX, ST. JAMES: Both make the authentic French versions.
- ARMY-NAVY STORE: For the real deal.

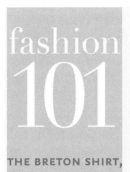

fashion 101

THE BRETON SHIRT, OR "THE MARINER"

The proper name for the striped sailor shirt is the Breton, since it originated in Brittany, France. In Brittany, seamen have been wearing these striped shirts since the 1820s. The original was made of very fine knit cotton and protected seamen from the wind and elements. The French Navy then made it part of the national uniform in 1858. It is thought that the prominent blue and white stripes served to more easily locate a man who had fallen into the sea. Let's face it, the shirt was meant to stand out even then.

84.
Suit

THE SUIT IS ALL ABOUT sleek sophistication. And though many men must wear one every day, women are allowed to pick and choose when they will don the item. This makes wearing one all the more striking. The trick is either to wear a lacy camisole underneath the suit jacket, or plain white tee, or nothing at all, and then play up the jewelry, hair, and makeup. And of course, pair the suit up with the perfect stilettos. These decidedly female touches let a woman own the suit, rather than having the suit own the woman.

My father used to say,
"Let them see you and not the suit—
that is secondary."

CARY GRANT

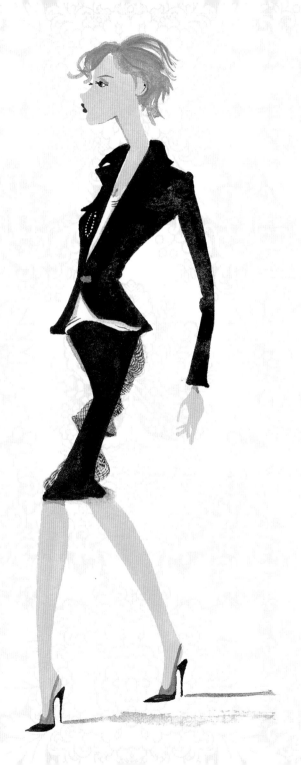

SUIT UP

- The cool, modern way to wear a suit is to break it up. Wear the jacket with jeans or the skirt with a tank or tee.
- As always, make sure it is tailored perfectly for you. Nothing beats great tailoring.
- When buying a suit for work, choose one that can work in a more fun way outside of the office. The double duty will truly be cost-effective for you in the long run.
- If you must wear a traditional suit to the office, personalize it with jewelry, etc. Always, always personalize it. Own it!

THE INSIDE TRACK: **WHERE TO BUY**

- Chanel is the timeless investment.
- Dolce & Gabbana and Alexander McQueen make the sexed-up versions.
- Ralph Lauren and Giorgio Armani are for the more classic look.

85.

Sunhat

A FLOPPY SUNHAT is a seaside staple, best found at roadside stands, flea markets, and beach-town shops. It is useful for keeping out the sun and/or hiding beachworn hair. It also lets the world know you are on holiday (even if you're not), especially when worn with a sundress and espadrilles. The sunhat is most often associated with carefree women who have nothing to do that day but smile. We should all aspire to be that woman, who looks like she has nothing to do but soak up the life around her.

HERE COMES THE SUN

- Michael Kors will often have a good version available.
- In general, the ultimate sunhat is bought on the fly at a roadside stand.
- It should pack easily—you are a girl on the go!

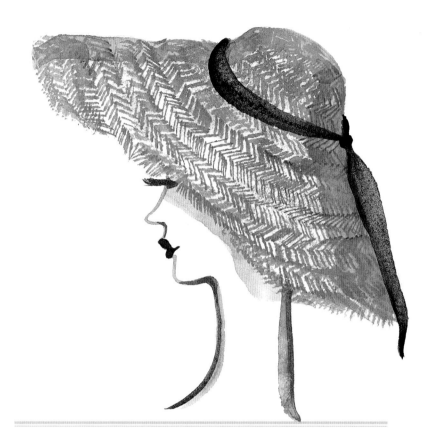

Live in the sunshine, swim in the sea,
drink the wild air.

RALPH WALDO EMERSON

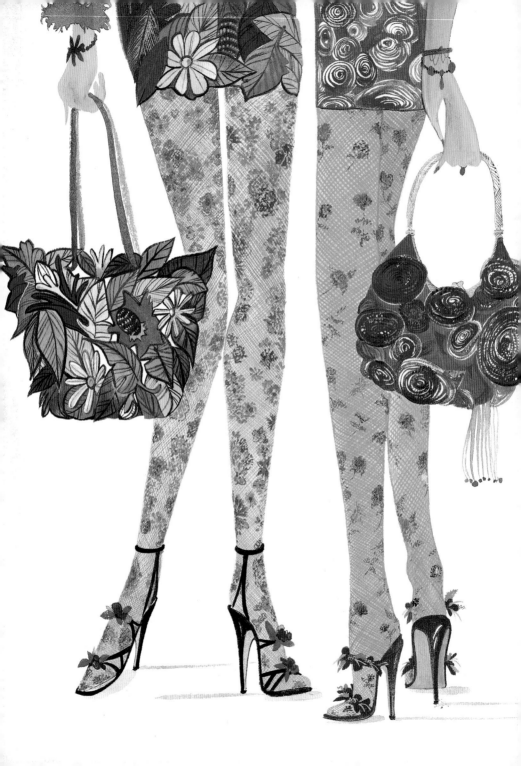

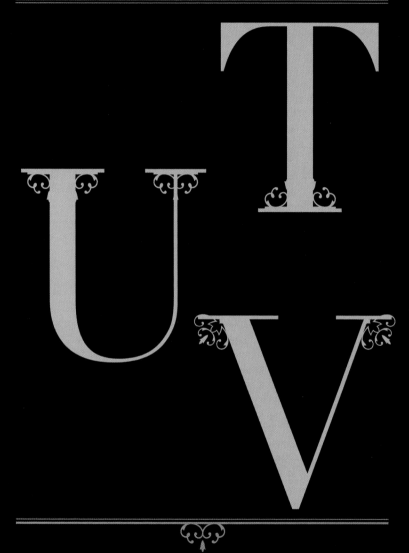

86.
Trench

———⬡⬡⬡———

WHEN YOU'VE GOT a great trench on, what's underneath isn't so important. Did you care what Catherine Deneuve was wearing under her Burberry in *The Umbrellas of Cherbourg*? I sure didn't. I was focused on the amazing coat, paired with only tights and a kitten heel. Ah, *l'amour!*

And in every film noir I've ever seen, I never cared what was underneath the coat the femme fatale wore. I barely even wanted the girl to take it off, because it seemed to be the only thing one should wear while going undercover. And perhaps it is because of these old films that the trench coat will always be an object of mystique. Whenever a girl feels like being a bit obscure, a bit inscrutable, a bit enigmatic, a trench coat is a must. Must! A great pair of sunglasses adds to the effect.

A fedora may be going a bit overboard, unless you are on the lam. But hey, a wanted girl has to do what a wanted girl has to do.

IN THE TRENCHES

Of course a khaki gabardine is the classic, but you can also dare to go for some edge, some color, or some gold lamé.

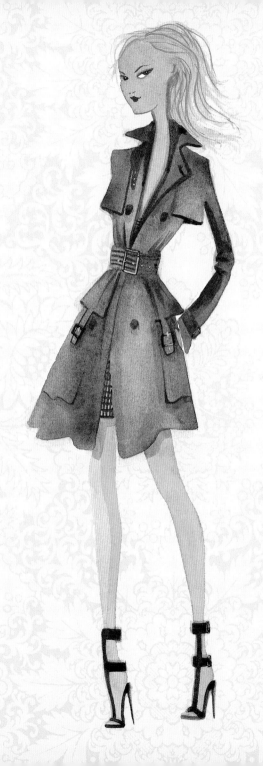

- FOR THE CLASSIC INVESTMENT: Burberry, of course.
- FOR AN EDGE: Look to Viktor & Rolf or Rock & Republic.
- FOR SOME COLOR: Juicy Couture or Gap.
- FOR METALLICS: Burberry (again) or Stella McCartney.

ICONIC TRENCH COAT WEARERS:

- Catherine Deneuve in *The Umbrellas of Cherbourg*
- Audrey Hepburn and George Peppard in *Breakfast at Tiffany's*
- Humphrey Bogart in *Casablanca*
- Meryl Streep in *Kramer vs. Kramer*
- Sophia Loren in *The Key*

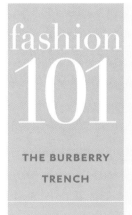

fashion
101

THE BURBERRY

TRENCH

Every aspect of the trench coat is purely functional, since it was originally created as a coat for British soldiers to wear during WWI. It is made of tightly woven gabardine, for water resistance. It is long enough to keep the rain out of a soldier's boots. It has a double-breasted closure and straps on the cuffs to tighten when it rains. When the soldiers returned home from war, they took their Burberrys with them and had them shortened for everyday wear. The coat became a British institution, a film-noir mainstay, and a style staple for both men and women since then.

87.
Turquoise and Coral Jewelry

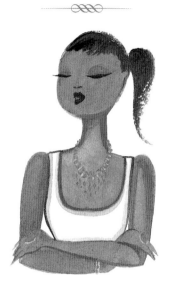

TURQUOISE IS one of those stones that you will often hear is "back," but as far as I'm concerned, it really never goes away. Is there not a season when a turquoise ring, necklace, or bracelet does not draw media attention or ravishing compliments? A turquoise Statement Necklace (#81) complements a Little White Dress (#49) and a summer tan every time. And during the winter, when everyone is in black and relying on plain gold jewelry, a few long strands of turquoise are going to make an outfit pop. In addition to turquoise being so chic, it also is said to have healing properties. It sure seems to make me feel better, every time I wear it.

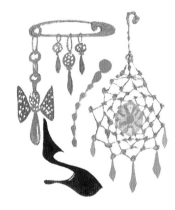

- Great when paired with coral, which is said to have the power to dispel the evil eye. When you wear your turquoise and coral together, you should be a formidable force.
- Turquoise seems to always say "summer," but because I love a broken rule, I think it looks quite amazing in the depths of winter, too.
- These pieces are wonderful to pick up when traveling in the American Southwest, Mexico, or India.
- Look for deep-colored turquoise. High-quality turquoise is opaque, while low quality is translucent.

FUN FACTS

- Turquoise jewelry dates back to 6000 BC.
- Turquoise is formed over millions of years, from water leaking through rocks containing minerals like copper and aluminum.
- Turquoise is a sacred stone for North American Indians and Tibetans, said to enhance mental and spiritual clarity, wisdom, trust, kindness, and understanding.

88.
Tuxedo Jacket

YOU MAY HAVE NOTICED that there are a fair number of items on this list that have been blatantly stolen from menswear, and that is for a good reason: Androgyny is forever chic and forever avant-garde. But it may have been Marlene Dietrich and her old tuxedo that really started the contemporary gender-bending style craze. The world was thrilled and/or scandalized. No woman had ever dared to wear men's clothes in such a blatant way. And in 1965, Yves Saint Laurent used the Marlene image to inspire his tuxedo jacket. With the forces of Marlene and YSL behind them, women began to enjoy the power that came with wearing a man's tuxedo jacket (tailored to fit the female frame, of course), and they were hooked. When photographer Helmut Newton captured Vibeke in YSL's tux in the 1970s, the craze (and that photo) were forever solidified in fashion history.

It is about style, not fashion.
Fashions come and go, but style is forever.

YVES SAINT LAURENT

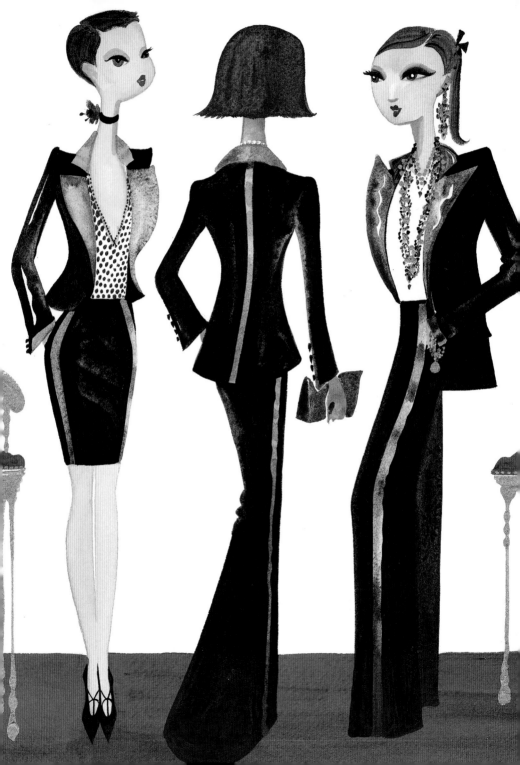

fashion 101

LE SMOKING

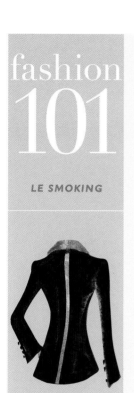

The tuxedo jacket is often referred to as *le smoking*, because of the original English term "smoking suit," referring to a suit intended for indoor use.

The tuxedo jacket was strictly men's property until 1966, when Yves Saint Laurent turned out a Spring/Summer collection that invited women into *le smoking* world. In a revolutionary-style instant, Saint Laurent sent his models down the runway in tuxedo jackets, turning the fashion world on its head. Overnight, he redefined the female silhouette and offered women a daring alternative to the little black dress. Countless style icons became instant and adoring fans: Catherine Deneuve, Betty Catroux, Françoise Hardy, Liza Minnelli, Loulou de la Falaise, Lauren Bacall, and Bianca Jagger.

YSL's tuxedo jacket made androgyny chic and elegant. It gave women a sense of power and changed the way they saw themselves. As Catherine Deneuve once said, "It really does make you feel different as a woman; it changes gestures."

NIP/TUX

- It should not fit like a man's tuxedo jacket, but rather should be slender and fit perfectly (see Blazer, #11).
- Try double-breasted if you are tall.
- Put a flower brooch on the lapel to work the androgyny in a really cool way.
- If you are feeling daring, don't wear anything underneath. Sexy.

89.

Umbrella

WEATHERMEN just cannot be trusted. They will tell you it's going to be a gorgeous and sunny day, and so you will happily and naively head out the door without an umbrella. Then, hours later, you and your perfectly blown-out head of hair are happily and naively walking down the street, and the skies open up to a not-so-gorgeous burst of rain. That moment is, in fact, apocalyptical. You are now probably cursing a weatherman's name. You are probably far from shelter. You are definitely wearing a white shirt. And the smarter girls are walking by with the mini umbrellas they keep at the bottom of their totes, and you are vowing to be one of those girls the next time your weatherman betrays you. A stylish woman is never caught off guard.

WHERE TO BUY . . .

- TOTES: Makes a mini one that fits in some of the smallest handbags made.
- BURBERRY: Makes the classic plaid version or a perfect all-black mini.

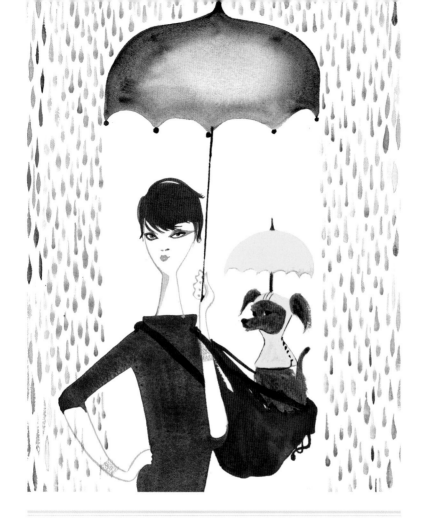

If you want the rainbow,
you've got to put up with the rain.

DOLLY PARTON

90.
Underwear

———⚬⚬⚬———

THE GAME BEGINS in the lingerie drawer. What you put on beneath your clothes matters. It's the basis for everything. It's amazing how quickly a great pair of underwear can make you feel sexy. And how quickly a bad panty line can ruin an outfit.

CLOSET OBSESSION: **UNDERCOVER AGENTS**

- Cosabella: Meaning "beautiful thing" in Italian. Cosabella is renowned for two things: comfort and color. The fan favorites are the Soire thongs, which come in over forty colors and counting. . . .
- OnGossamer: Beloved by celebrities, the OnGossamer invisible mesh boy shorts are the perfect option for those who are not G-string fans.
- La Perla: The famed Italian lingerie company makes seamless and luxurious thongs, hipsters, and culottes.
- Elle Macpherson Intimates: Knickers from a woman who knows a thing or two about underwear (and style). These pieces are playful, sensual, and flat-out fashionable.

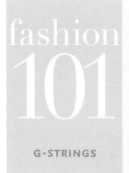

fashion 101

G-STRINGS

G-strings are the oldest form of clothing known to man. They have been worn by tribal peoples for over 75,000 years. The G-string was originally designed for men, and it only came to be worn as an undergarment for Western women in the 1980s.

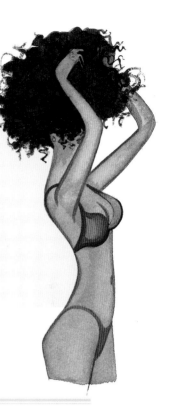

My mother was right.
When you've got nothing left
all you can do is get into some silk underwear
and start reading Proust.

JANE BIRKIN

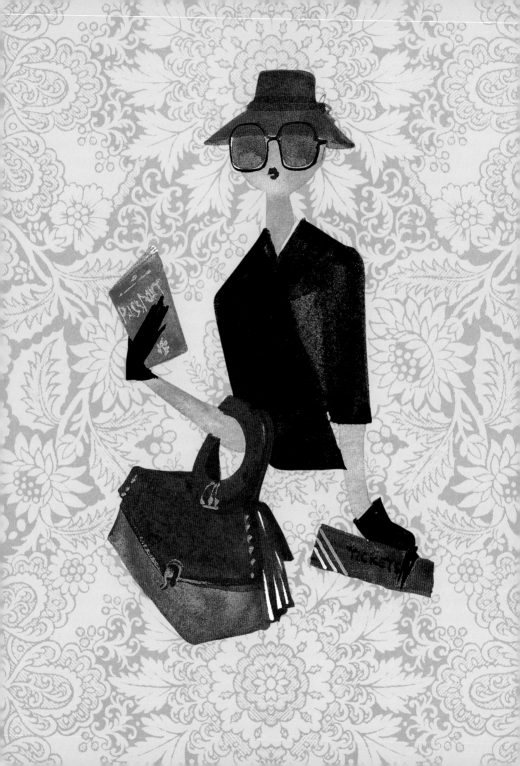

91.
Valid Passport

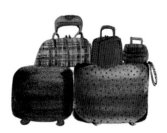

IT IS ALWAYS TWO WEEKS before you are leaving on a trip when you realize that your passport expired last month. Or when you realize you have no idea where you've placed the damn thing. You are going to be sitting in that passport office and/or using a rush service for renewal, which costs way too much money and will seriously cut into your shopping funds. Don't let this ever happen to you!

You can get a fabulous passport case from Vuitton, Goyard, or Hermès in an exotic skin. It's an affordable item from a high-end brand and will make you feel glamorous and somewhat ameliorate the horror that air travel has become.

Adventure is worthwhile in itself.

AMELIA EARHART

92.

Vans

THERE IS a continental divide between Converse and Vans. The East Coast says Converse, the West Coast says Vans. Why not both? Vans are the sneakers to wear when looking California cool. The added benefit of Vans is that the company lets you customize sneakers so they can be uniquely yours.

SKATER CHIC

- Definitely go for the customized option. Be unique—Golden Rule.
- Wear them with supercasual dresses in summer for the ultimate California Girl look.
- Use them to instantly add street cred to the stuffiest outfit (see Suit, #84).

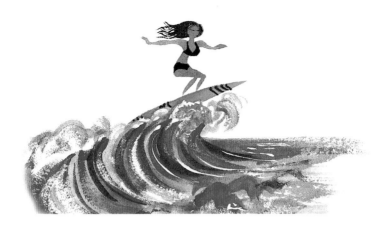

fashion
101

VANS

Vans were created in the '60s and are a SoCal legend. It was the West Coast skating community that earned the company a cultish following. Skaters in Manhattan Beach and Santa Monica began entering stores and asking for custom-made pairs (the company is famous for its customized services), and soon every skater (and surfer) along the California coast had a pair of Vans. Then, in the 1980s, Vans hit the big time when a little movie called *Fast Times at Ridgemont High* hit the theaters. Spicoli (Sean Penn) wore his pair of checkered Vans everywhere, and within weeks the company was producing millions of pairs of the shoe.

All I need are some tasty waves,
a cool buzz, and I'm fine.

JEFF SPICOLI IN *FAST TIMES AT RIDGEMONT HIGH*

93.
Vintage

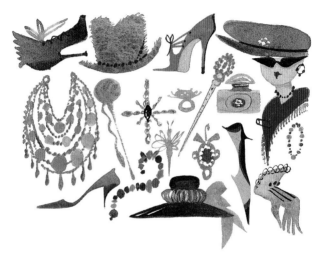

VINTAGE ITEMS ARE a fantastic way to add individual style to a wardrobe and set yourself apart from the pack. Nobody is going to have that same dress or coat you got from the local thrift shop. Nobody. The other advantage of buying vintage is that you can find a lot of designer items at bargain-bin prices. If you know your fashion history, you'll know the labels and items to look out for (a YSL tuxedo jacket, a Courrèges A-line, a Pucci or Missoni print). However, there are definite pitfalls when buying vintage. One must definitely be aware of these pitfalls, for falling into one can make you go from chic to cheap in no time.

THE KEY WHEN BUYING VINTAGE
IS TO BE STRICT

- The condition should be perfect. No pulling, stains, or discoloration. This is the difference between looking fab or looking shabby.
- The garment should fit, or at least it should be big enough so that you can tailor it to fit. Never buy too small.
- A vintage designer dress can be found for much less if you know who to look for—Missoni, Pucci, Alaia.
- It is best to start your vintage journey in the accessories section. You generally cannot go wrong with vintage jewelry or clutches.

THE INSIDE TRACK:
A FEW FAVORITE VINTAGE SHOPS

- Los Angeles: Decades, Paper Bag Princess
- New York: What Goes Around Comes Around
- Miami: Rags to Riches
- Chicago: The Daisy Shop
- Boston: Second Time Around

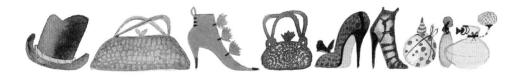

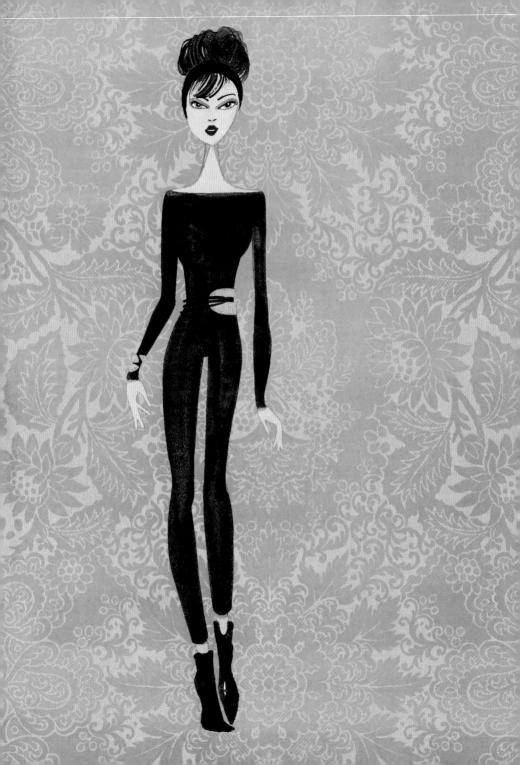

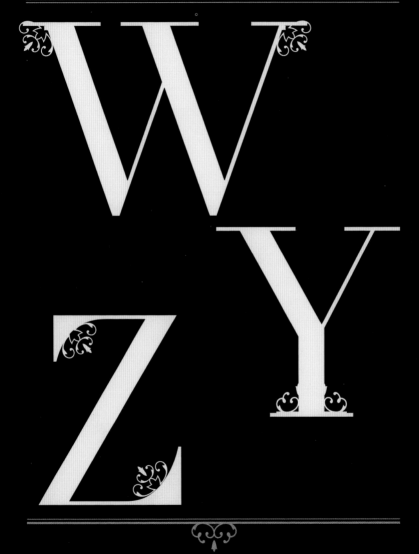

94

Watch

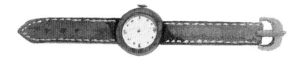

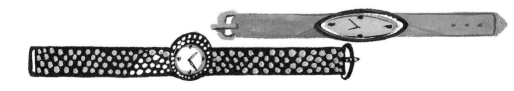

NOW THAT MOST OF US KNOW what time it is by looking at our cell phones, we no longer have to wear a
watch for practical reasons. Watches have become
pure fashion items and should serve as statement
pieces rather than timepieces. There are a few ways
to go with a watch, depending on your personality, sensibility, and
current shopping fund. You can go really feminine and high-end
and get a diamond cocktail watch (a gorgeous investment if you can
swing it). You can go trendy and get the newest plastic watch from
Prada or Swatch. You be a classicist and get a timeless silver design
(be it Rolex or TAG Heuer). Or you can opt for a man's watch. I personally love the look of a man's watch on a woman's wrist. The big,
bold masculinity of the design draws the eye to the wrist, one of the
most feminine parts of a woman's body.

INSIDE TRACK: **MY FAVORITES**

These are my favorite three iconic watches. They are all break-the-bank pieces—because, hey, a watch should be a break-the-bank item.

- Cartier Tank: The Cartier Tank was created in 1917, at the height of World War I, and legend has it that Louis Cartier based the design on the horizontal section of the Renault military tank. It dramatically changed the history of watches; due to its popularity, it inspired men and women to switch from pocket watches to wristwatches. Over the years, there have been over 250 variations on the original Cartier Tank.
- Rolex Daytona: In 1961, Rolex released this chronograph (a watch with both timekeeping and stopwatch features), and it was instantly a favorite watch of race car drivers, since it could be used to easily calculate lap speed. It was soon named the Daytona, after the popular Florida racetrack. Due to its limited production (from 1961 to 1987) and unlimited popularity, the Daytona is one of the most coveted and collectible watches.
- Jaeger-LeCoultre Reverso: It was created in 1931, and it is so named because of its reversible swivel case. It was made for English Army officers in India, who frequently broke their wristwatch crystals while playing polo. Jaeger-LeCoultre produced a case that could turn 180 degrees, and therefore the crystal is not exposed when playing polo . . . or in the trenches of a sample sale.

95.
Wayfarers

R AY-BAN WAYFARERS have been worn by everyone from Kim Novak to Mary-Kate Olsen, Bob Dylan to Chloë Sevigny. They were created in 1952 and exploited the new plastics technology of the era. The distinctive trapezoidal frames and sturdy arms were aimed to make the sunglasses look masculine, since it was originally thought to be a man's sunglass. But in 1954, when Kim Novak wore them on the Côte d'Azur, it was clearly not going to be just a man's sunglass any longer. Though they were popular with the men—John Lennon, Roy Orbison—it was good old Audrey Hepburn (my Goddess) who made the Wayfarers seem so utterly feminine when she wore them in *Breakfast at Tiffany's*. In the '60s, when the movie came out, every girl had to have a pair. The Wayfarer went in and out of vogue for a few decades, but it always came back with a vengeance. Now that we are more than a half-century away from the inception of the Wayfarer, I think it's safe to say that they are an item that is not going away.

SHADY CHARACTERS

- 1961: Audrey Hepburn in *Breakfast at Tiffany's*
- 1980: John Belushi and Dan Aykroyd in *The Blues Brothers*
- 1983: Tom Cruise in *Risky Business*
- 1984–89: Don Johnson in *Miami Vice*
- 1985: Madonna in *Desperately Seeking Susan*

WAYFARERING . . .

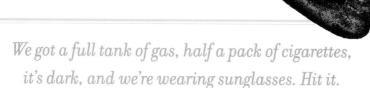

- The red- and white-framed versions have their moments, but the black is the ultimate model.
- Those big, bold, incognito sunglasses will come and go, but the Wayfarers will never make you look like a fashion victim.

We got a full tank of gas, half a pack of cigarettes,
it's dark, and we're wearing sunglasses. Hit it.

THE BLUES BROTHERS

96.
Wellington Boot

WHEN KATE MOSS showed up at the Glastonbury Music Festival in 2005, she was wearing a barely there gold lamé dress and a pair of black Hunter Wellingtons. The photos of her sloshing around in the mud were seen around the world (we all still remember the image, I'm sure), and afterward, women everywhere pulled out their Wellingtons, realizing they were kind of cool. Women began to wear their Wellies with dresses, skirts, or skinny jeans. Rain or shine. Of course, the Wellie remains the most practical option for times of rain. And when attending music festivals, they now seem the *only* option.

CLOSET OBSESSION: **HUNTERS**

Hunters are a UK institution. Every Brit has at least one pair in his or her closet, and the Royal Family always wears the classic green version for mucking about in the country. Because of their comfort and practicality, Wellies have become more than just a UK institution. Women around the world eagerly order Wellies (and the ones who know what they are doing know to order a size down from what they usually wear—they run big).

In the early 1800s, the first Duke of Wellington asked his shoemaker to modify the Hessian boot to be durable for battle but comfortable enough for evening. The shoemaker came up with the design for the Wellington boot. The first boots were made of leather until 1852, when the Hunter Company began to make them of rubber.

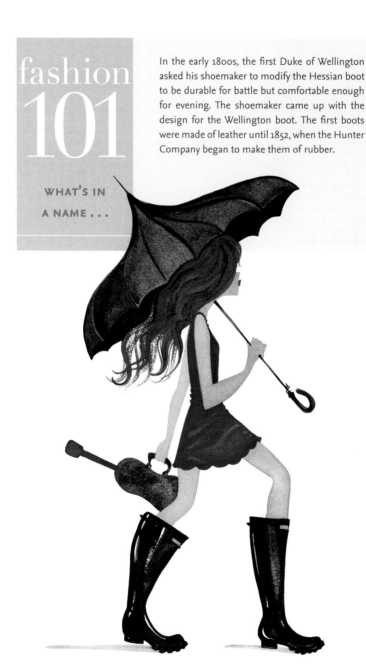

97.
Wide-Leg Trousers

W E OWE a debt of gratitude to Katharine Hepburn for the wide-leg trouser. They offer freedom of movement and are glamorous. A combination that is rare indeed. The story goes that in 1938, when she was filming *Bringing Up Baby*, Hepburn continually wore pants on set. When the executives asked her to stop, she refused. Then one day, her trousers disappeared from her dressing room. Katharine, unruffled, walked around the set in her underwear, until her pants were returned. Katharine, along with Marlene Dietrich (see Tuxedo Jacket, #88) were the forerunners in setting down what garments to steal from the men . . . and how to never let men steal those items back from you.

I like to move fast, and wearing high heels was tough, and low heels with a skirt is unattractive.

So pants took over.

KATHARINE HEPBURN

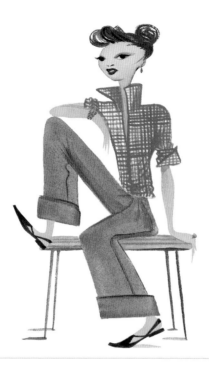

WIDE-EYED

- Only wear wide-legged styles with something fitted on top, to balance off the bulk on bottom.
- Look for a pair with a cuff, and leave the hemline a little long—too short is not a good look!
- A flat front is more flattering than pleats.
- Be careful of pocket placement—you don't want flaps on your hips, otherwise it will widen instead of slim your hips.
- Try them in black, white, camel, or pinstripe for the most enduring styles.

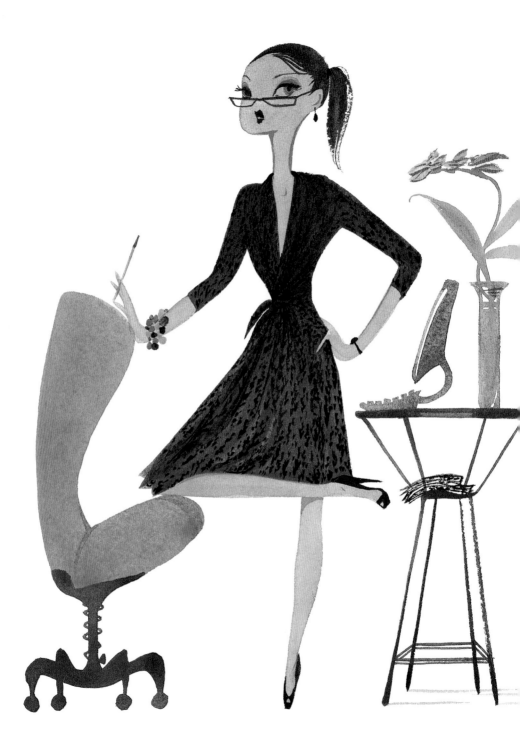

98.
Wrap Dress

⸙

I N THE '70S, Diane Von Furstenberg made the wrap into the ultimate dress for women of all shapes and sizes. If there is one dress designed with the intention of flattering the woman's figure, it is the wrap dress. It hugs all the right places and elegantly drapes over the others. And the waist-cinching sash allows us to play around with it until the fit is just right. We can be our own tailor each time we wear it. When wearing the wrap dress, be your own daring stylist, as the dress is a timeless piece meant to be creatively toyed with.

IT'S A WRAP!

· Buy it in jersey, the original fabric of the dress, as it is the best fabric for curve-enhanced hugging.
· Buy it in a print to give it a bit of flair. It's a timeless dress, so the print and colors can be as outlandish as you want.
· Try wearing it with boots or stilettos, and maybe even consider wearing it with jeans. Point is, try it with everything.

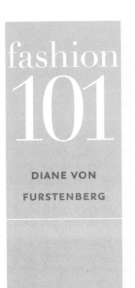

fashion
101

DIANE VON FURSTENBERG

In the '70s, Diane Von Furstenberg was working in a little factory and started experimenting with jersey and little wrap dancer tops. Then she had the idea to make the tops into full dresses, and the idea took off. In 1975, she sold five million of her wrap dresses and landed on the cover of *Newsweek* and the *Wall Street Journal*. "I design for the woman who loves being a woman," she said, and you can tell by the form and function of the wrap dress that she absolutely believes this. Every aspect serves to enhance a woman's body. In the early '80s, she stopped designing and focused on several other ventures (cosmetics, for one), but in 1997 she came back to us, and now we don't have to fight over the invaluable vintage finds (though I still will if I see one I have to have).

Life is a risk.

DIANE VON FURSTENBERG

99.
Yoga Gear

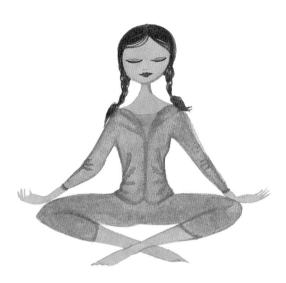

N O INNER PEACE was ever achieved in a baggy sweat-shirt and old sweatpants. Workout clothes should fit you just as well as your street clothes. If your gym clothes are old, stretched, or faded, replace them! You deserve to look good in those gym mirrors—after all, you did make it to the gym (a victory in and of itself), so you'd better have some nice clothes to stretch and sweat in since you're there. Just promise not to wear them on an airplane. (It's often assumed that nice yoga clothes or even a nice sweatsuit can be worn on a plane. That is a total mistake.)

NUALA AND MAHANUALA

Nuala (an acronym for *Natural Universal Altruistic Limitless Authentic*) is a line of yoga clothes by Christy Turlington in collaboration with Puma. The clothes are not just yoga-friendly, they are stylish enough to wear on the street without being embarrassing (we would expect nothing less from the supermodel). A second line, Mahanuala, also by Christy, was created in 2004, and has more items for the serious Yogi. Christy said that she created the lines out of need, because every other brand on the market was using synthetic materials and outlandish colors.

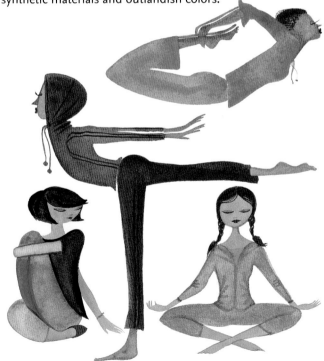

100.
Zippered Hoodie

───────⊗⊗⊗───────

THE ZIPPERED HOODIE has become the denim or leather jacket of the modern day. Once an item worn exclusively by the fringe, it is now clearly within fashion territory. It seems that every respectable celebrity, musician, and model owns at least twenty of these. They are mandatory for going through the corridors of JFK, Hollywood Boulevard, and Saturday morning Starbucks runs. But when it is stepped up to a cashmere or fine merino wool version, it becomes a grown-up item that can be worn on the most sophisticated of occasions.

IN THE HOOD

- Make sure your hoodie is fitted so that you look sleek and fashionable, not sloppy and frumpy.
- Always keep the hood up when your hair is less than perfect and there are paparazzi around.
- Buy a black cashmere version! (If I leave you with one last tip, it is to *always* buy a black cashmere version of an item if it comes in a black cashmere version.)

The first hooded sweatshirt was made by Champion and was created to keep laborers warm in the frozen warehouses of New York. It took off as a fashion item in the '70s, when hip-hop was gaining ground and the hoodie was the subculture's uniform of choice. It also achieved a huge boost in 1976, when Sylvester Stallone appeared onscreen in his trademark *Rocky* hoodie. Over the decades, the hoodie became the standard garment of choice for the young, the brooding, and the cooler-than-thou (i.e., skater boys, punk rockers, the hip-hop crowd, surfer dudes, paparazzi-avoiding celebrities).

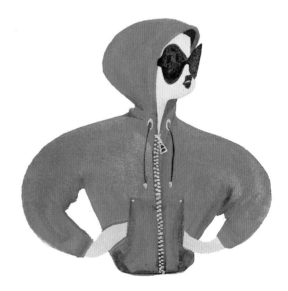

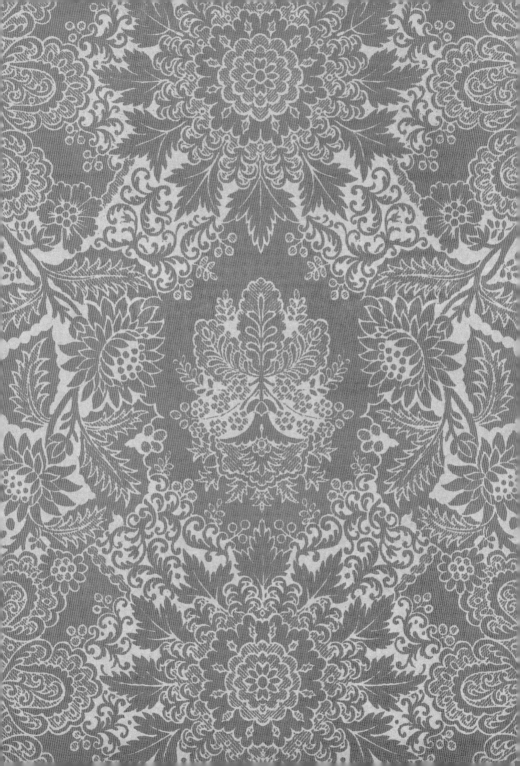

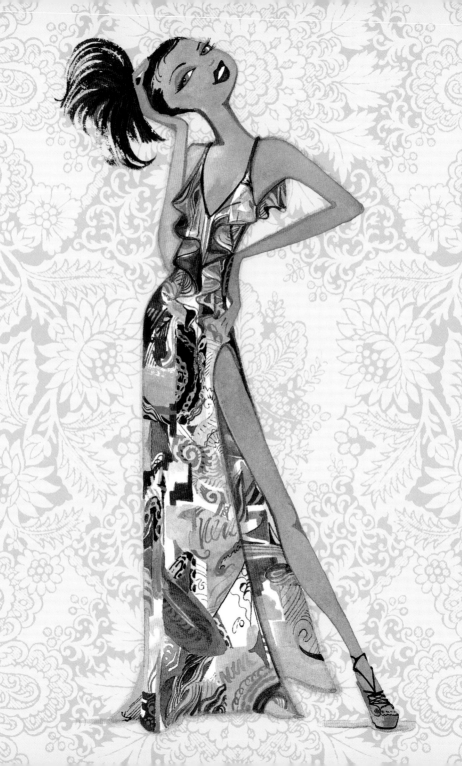

Parting Words . . .

TODAY'S FASHION CYCLES are getting shorter and frighteningly fast. There are more trends and more choices, and it seems that we are always under pressure to keep up. Calm down. Do not be moved by these fashion distractions. Do not be the woman who gets caught up in the fads. You should be the woman who has a personal style and who is not afraid to wear your favorite one hundred pieces repeatedly (while mixing in a few fads here and there for fun). Remember, repetition is a sign of style. There is a name for the women who wear a new outfit every single day: fashion victims.

When you change your look so many times, it seems like you are confused. You also deny yourself any chance of developing a trademark style. Yet, when you invest deeply in pieces that you love and will love season after season, these items become *yours*. And when you wear these items over and over again—your mother's heirloom necklace, your old Chanel jacket, your favorite black dress—they become a part of you. They show the world that you know who you are. You are no fashion victim. You are an original. Start dressing like one.

Nina

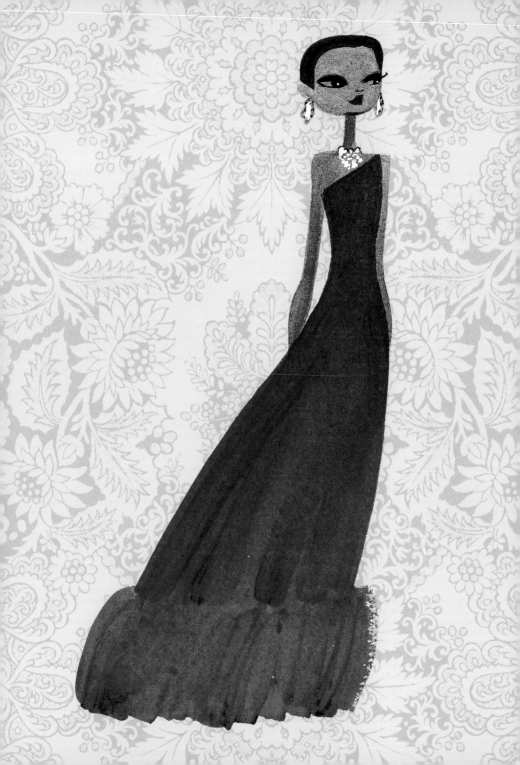

Acknowledgments

A THANK YOU TO my family and all my friends for their constant inspiration and support. I'm blessed to be surrounded by a network of truly the most talented and intelligent people one could imagine.

Ruben Toledo, for his magnificent illustrations. His talent is a global treasure. Every detail is a work of art and I am honored to have my name printed alongside his. And, of course, Isabel Toledo, the woman beside the man (and always sporting the most fabulous of chic items—she's the embodiment of *The One Hundred*).

Rene Alegria, for his infectious creative zeal. This book would never have come to be without him, his patience, and his gentle (but firm!) guidance.

Marissa Matteo, who is an absolute blast to work with. She helped make the process as smooth as possible, and her eclectic brain is a marvel to witness in action.

Shubhani Sarkar is a genius. Period. She has an aesthetic gift and spirit that, if she were in fashion, would be the envy of all.

Everyone at HarperCollins for their endless days of work to make this book what it is. In particular, the talented Melinda Moore, Amy Vreeland, Grace Veras, Susan Kosko, Lorie Pagnozzi, Carla Clifford, Angie Lee, Felicia Sullivan, Samantha Hagerbaumer, Janina Mak, Andrea Rosen, Paul Olsewski, Michelle Dominguez, Doug Jones, Margot Schupf, Mary Ellen O'Neill, and Steve Ross.

David and Lucas Conrod, for being so great to come home to . . . and for giving me endless excuses to go to the park. They are my real inspiration.

Everyone at *Project Runway*, all of the PR contestants, Bravo, Lifetime, and The Weinstein Company, for making the show such a huge success.

And finally, the fashion industry, with its unlimited beauty and possibilities. I believe in what I do, in who we are. Nothing will ever let me lose sight of this.

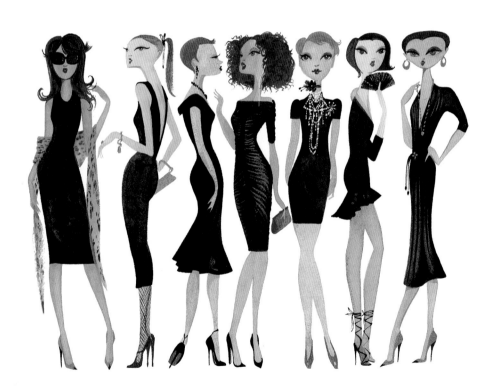